POCKET GUIDE TO
Chronic Kidney Disease and the Nutrition Care Process

SECOND EDITION

Jessie M. Pavlinac
MS, RDN-AP, CSR, LD, FNKF, FAND

Arianna Aoun
MS, RDN, LD

Academy of Nutrition and Dietetics
Chicago, IL

Academy of Nutrition and Dietetics

Academy of Nutrition and Dietetics
120 S. Riverside Plaza, Suite 2190
Chicago, IL 60606

Academy of Nutrition and Dietetics Pocket Guide to Chronic Kidney Disease and the Nutrition Care Process, Second Edition

ISBN 978-0-88091-228-0 (print)
ISBN 978-0-88091-229-7 (eBook)
Catalog Number 479324 (print)
Catalog Number 479324e (eBook)

Copyright © 2024, Academy of Nutrition and Dietetics. All rights reserved. Except for brief quotations embodied in critical articles or reviews, no part of this publication may be reproduced, stored in a retrieval system, or transmitted, in any form or by any means, electronic, mechanical, photocopying, recording, or otherwise, without the prior written consent of the publisher.

The views expressed in this publication are those of the authors and do not necessarily reflect policies and/or official positions of the Academy of Nutrition and Dietetics. Mention of product names in this publication does not constitute endorsement by the authors or the Academy of Nutrition and Dietetics. The Academy of Nutrition and Dietetics disclaims responsibility for the application of the information contained herein.

10 9 8 7 6 5 4 3 2 1

For more information on the Academy of Nutrition and Dietetics, visit www.eatright.org.

Library of Congress Cataloging-in-Publication Data

Names: Pavlinac, Jessie M., author. | Aoun, Arianna, author.
Title: Pocket guide to chronic kidney disease and the nutrition care
  process / editors, Jessie M. Pavlinac, MS, RDN-AP, CSR, LD, FNKF, FAND,
  Arianna Aoun, MS, RDN, LD.
Description: Second edition. | Chicago, IL : Academy of Nutrition and
  Dietetics, [2023] | Includes bibliographical references and index.
Identifiers: LCCN 2023028289 (print) | LCCN 2023028290 (ebook) | ISBN
  9780880912280 (spiral bound) | ISBN 9780880912297 (ebook)
Subjects: LCSH: Chronic renal failure--Nutritional aspects. |
  Kidneys--Diseases--Nutritional aspects. |
  Kidneys--Diseases--Patients--Nutrition.
Classification: LCC RC918.R4 P38 2023 (print) | LCC RC918.R4 (ebook) |
  DDC 616.6/14--dc23/eng/20230710
LC record available at https://lccn.loc.gov/2023028289
LC ebook record available at https://lccn.loc.gov/2023028290

Contents

List of Boxes, Tables, and Figures iv

Frequently Used Terms and Abbreviations viii

Reviewers xv

Preface xvi

Acknowledgments xvii

About the Authors xviii

Publisher's Note on Gender-Inclusive Language xx

Chapter 1: Chronic Kidney Disease, Evidence-Based Practice, and the Nutrition Care Process 1

Chapter 2: Nutrition Assessment 15

Chapter 3: Nutrition Diagnosis 54

Chapter 4: Nutrition Intervention—Part 1: Planning the Nutrition Prescription 70

Chapter 5: Nutrition Intervention—Part 2: Implementation 133

Chapter 6: Nutrition Monitoring and Evaluation 169

Appendix: Commonly Prescribed Renal-Specific Vitamins 184

Continuing Professional Education 187

Index 188

List of Boxes, Tables, and Figures

Boxes

Box 1.1 Steps of the Nutrition Care Process 4

Box 1.2 Strength of Recommendation and Quality of Evidence 7

Box 1.3 Medicare Conditions for Coverage Mandates Related to the Nutrition Care Process and Documentation 9

Box 2.1 Food/Nutrition-Related Data Needed to Perform an Assessment 16

Box 2.2 Antihypertensive Medications Used in Chronic Kidney Disease 19

Box 2.3 Phosphate-Binding Medications Used in Chronic Kidney Disease 22

Box 2.4 Hypoglycemic Agents Used in Chronic Kidney Disease 27

Box 2.5 Dosing Adjustments for Medicines Used to Treat Lipid Disorders in Chronic Kidney Disease 29

Box 2.6 Possible Effects of Selected Drugs on Nutrient Absorption and Utilization 30

Box 2.7 International Classification of Adult Weight According to BMI 33

Box 2.8 Proposed Mechanisms for the Association of Obesity With Chronic Kidney Disease 34

Box 2.9 Biochemical Data Used in Nutrition Assessment of
Patients With Chronic Kidney Disease 35

Box 2.10 Interpretation of Biochemical Data in Chronic
Kidney Disease 37

Box 2.11 Calculating Ideal, Standard, and Adjusted Body Weight
in Patients With Chronic Kidney Disease 45

Box 3.1 Selected Intake Domain Nutrition Diagnoses for Chronic
Kidney Disease 57

Box 3.2 Selected Clinical Domain Nutrition Diagnoses for Chronic
Kidney Disease 59

Box 3.3 Selected Behavioral-Environmental Domain Nutrition
Diagnoses for Chronic Kidney Disease 61

Box 4.1 Considerations in Developing a Nutrition Prescription
for Chronic Kidney Disease 71

Box 4.2 The Metabolically Stable Patient 76

Box 4.3 Recommended Micronutrients for Patients With
Chronic Kidney Disease, Not on Dialysis 82

Box 4.4 Suggested Composition of Parenteral Nutrition
Solution for Adults With Chronic Kidney Disease 89

Box 4.5 Maintenance Hemodialysis and Peritoneal Dialysis
Medical Nutrition Therapy Recommendations 93

Box 4.6 Long-Chain Omega-3 Polyunsaturated Fatty Acids
in the Adult Dialysis Population 97

Box 4.7 Daily Vitamin Recommendations for Hemodialysis 100

Box 4.8 Macronutrient and Electrolyte Considerations in
Intradialytic Parenteral Nutrition 109

Box 4.9 Nutrition Guidelines for Nocturnal Hemodialysis
Administered at Home 112

Box 4.10 Acute-Phase Medical Nutrition Therapy
After Kidney Transplant 114

Box 4.11 Chronic-Phase Medical Nutrition Therapy After
Kidney Transplant 115

Box 5.1 Phosphorus Supplementation 134

Box 5.2 Oral Supplements and Enteral Formulas for
Chronic Kidney Disease 136

Box 5.3 Nutrition Education Resources for Chronic
Kidney Disease 140

Box 5.4 Physical Activity Guidelines 142

Box 5.5 Appetite Stimulants and Their Adverse Effects 142

Box 5.6 Components and Principles of Diabetes and Chronic
Kidney Disease Self-Management 146

Box 5.7 Potential Nutrition-Related Adverse Effects of
Immunosuppressants and Possible Interventions 149

Box 5.8 Food Safety Recommendations for Immunosuppressed
Individuals 151

Box 5.9 Motivational Interviewing Techniques 153

Box 5.10 Transtheoretical Model of Intentional Behavior Change
(Stages of Change) 155

Box 5.11 Strategies for Modifying Behavior 157

Box 5.12 Strategies for Maintaining Behavior Change 158

Box 6.1 Nutrition Monitoring and Evaluation Recommendations 171

Box 6.2 Recommended Measures for Monitoring Nutritional
Status of Patients on Maintenance Dialysis Annually or
When Status Change Indicates 172

Box 6.3 Key Nutrition Care Process–Related Charting Elements
for Medical Records 173

Tables

Table 1.1 Stages of Chronic Kidney Disease 3

Table 1.2 Medicare Part B Reimbursement for Medical Nutrition
Therapy for Patients With Chronic Kidney Disease 5

Table 2.1 Frequency of Measures to Evaluate Metabolic Bone
Disease in Patients With Chronic Kidney Disease 43

Table 2.2 Amputation Adjustments 46

Table 2.3 Suggested Adjustment Factors for Estimating
Energy Needs 47

Table 4.1 Medical Nutrition Therapy Recommendations for Chronic
Kidney Disease Stages 1 Through 5, Not on Dialysis, With
or Without Diabetes 72

Table 4.2 Commercially Available Oral Ketoacid/Amino
Acid Analogs 77

Table 4.3 Sample Parenteral Nutrition Formulations 88

Table 4.4 Sample Intravenous Fat Emulsions for Parenteral Nutrition 89

Table 4.5 Dextrose Contribution of Peritoneal Dialysis Solutions 96

Table 4.6 Phosphorus Absorption From Various Diet Sources 104

Table 4.7 Comparison of Hemodialysis Treatment Times 111

Table 5.1 National Renal Diet Exchanges for Chronic
Kidney Disease 145

Table 5.2 Common Oral Iron Supplements 148

Figures

Figure 3.1 Common nutrition diagnoses in my practice 64

Frequently Used Terms and Abbreviations

5D	CKD stage 5, on dialysis
5ND	CKD stage 5, not on dialysis
AA	amino acids
AAKP	American Association of Kidney Patients
ABW	adjusted body weight
ACE	angiotensin-converting enzyme (inhibitors)
ADIME	assessment, diagnosis, intervention, monitoring and evaluation
ADLs	activities of daily living
AKI	acute kidney injury
Alb	albumin
Alk Phos	alkaline phosphatase
APD	ambulatory peritoneal dialysis
ARB	angiotensin receptor blocker
ASN	American Society of Nephrology
ASPEN	American Society for Parenteral and Enteral Nutrition
AV	arteriovenous
BEE	basal energy expenditure
BUN	blood urea nitrogen
BW	body weight

Ca	calcium
CaCO$_3$	calcium carbonate
CAPD	continuous ambulatory peritoneal dialysis
CBG	capillary blood glucose
CCPD	continuous cyclic peritoneal dialysis
CfC	Conditions for Coverage (from CMS)
CHr	reticulocyte hemoglobin content
CKD	chronic kidney disease
CKD-EPI	Chronic Kidney Disease Epidemiology Collaboration
CKD-MBD	chronic kidney disease-mineral and bone disorder
CMS	Centers for Medicare & Medicaid Services
cm	centimeters
CO$_2$	carbon dioxide
Cr	creatinine
CRP	C-reactive protein
CRRT	continuous renal replacement therapy
D	Dialysis
d	day
DASH	Dietary Approaches to Stop Hypertension (diet)
DFO	deferoxamine
DHHS	Department of Health and Human Services
DKD	diabetic kidney disease
dL	deciliter
DM	diabetes mellitus
DRI	Dietary Reference Intake
DSM	*Diagnostic and Statistical Manual of Mental Disorders*

EAL	Evidence Analysis Library (of the Academy of Nutrition and Dietetics)
EBNPG	evidence-based nutrition practice guidelines
EDW	estimated dry weight
eGFR	estimated glomerular filtration rate
eNCPT	electronic Nutrition Care Process Terminology
ESA	erythropoiesis-stimulating agent
ESKD	end-stage kidney disease
ESRD	end-stage renal disease
Fe	iron
g	gram
GFR	glomerular filtration rate
GI	gastrointestinal
Glofil	glomerular filtration
GRADE	Grading Recommendations Assessment, Development, and Evaluation
h	hour
HCl	hydrochloride
HD	hemodialysis
HDL	high-density lipoprotein
Hgb	hemoglobin
HbA1c	hemoglobin A1c
HMG CoA	β-hydroxy β-methylglutaryl-CoA (reductase inhibitors)
HTN	hypertension
IADLs	instrumental activities of daily living
IBW	ideal body weight
ICU	intensive care unit

Frequently Used Terms and Abbreviations

IDPN	intradialytic parenteral nutrition
IDWG	interdialytic weight gain
IG	interpretive guideline
IHD	intermittent hemodialysis
IPAA	intraperitoneal amino acid
iPTH	intact parathyroid hormone
IU	international unit
IV	intravenous
IVF	intravenous fluid
K	potassium
KA	ketoacid
KDIGO	Kidney Disease: Improving Global Outcomes
KDOQI	Kidney Disease Outcomes Quality Initiative
LC	long chain
LDL	low-density lipoprotein
LEE	lower-extremity edema
LLC	limited liability corporation
MAC	microalbumin-to-creatinine ratio
MCH	mean corpuscular hemoglobin
MCT	medium chain triglyceride
MCV	mean corpuscular volume
MEI	Medical Education Institute
mEq	milliequivalent
Mg	magnesium
MHD	maintenance hemodialysis
MIS	Malnutrition Inflammation Score
MNT	medical nutrition therapy

MUFA	monounsaturated fatty acids
MVI	multivitamin
n-3	omega 3
Na	sodium
NCEP	National Cholesterol Education Program
NCP	Nutrition Care Process
NCPM	Nutrition Care Process and Model
NCPT	Nutrition Care Process Terminology
NEAP	net acid production
NFPF	nutrition focused physical findings
NHANES II	National Health and Nutrition Examination Survey II
NHD	nocturnal hemodialysis
NHHD	nocturnal home hemodialysis
NIDDK	National Institute of Diabetes and Digestive and Kidney Diseases
NIH	National Institutes of Health
NKDEP	National Kidney Disease Education Program
NKF	National Kidney Foundation
NKF-ASN	National Kidney Foundation-American Society of Nephrology
NKP-CRN	National Kidney Foundation-Council on Renal Nutrition
NKF-KDOQI	National Kidney Foundation-Kidney Disease Outcomes Quality Initiative
NLM	National Library of Medicine
NODAT	new-onset diabetes after transplantation
nPNA	normalized protein nitrogen appearance
ONS	oral nutrition supplements

OTC	over-the-counter
PA	physical activity
PD	peritoneal dialysis
PES	problem, etiology, signs and symptoms
PEW	protein energy wasting
PN	parenteral nutrition
PO	by mouth
PO_4	phosphorus
POC	plan of care
PPN	peripheral parenteral nutrition
PPS	Prospective Payment System
PTH	parathyroid hormone
PUFA	polyunsaturated fatty acids
QoL	quality of life
RBC	red blood cell
RDA	Recommended Dietary Allowance
RDN	registered dietitian nutritionist
RPG	Renal Practice Group
RRT	renal replacement therapy
Rx	prescription
SGA	subjective global assessment
s-Ca	serum calcium
s-K	serum potassium
$s\text{-}PO_4$	serum phosphorus
TG	triglycerides
TIBC	total iron-binding capacity
TID	three times a day

TSAT	transferrin saturation (ratio of serum iron to total iron binding capacity)
U/L	units per liter
VLDL	very low-density lipoprotein
WBC	white blood count
WNL	within normal limits

Reviewers

Julie Driscoll, RDN, CSR
Dietitian and Health Services Administrator,
Department of Justice, Federal Bureau of Prisons
Ayer, MA

Rosa K. Hand, PhD, RDN, LD, FAND
Professor, Nutrition, Case Western Reserve University
Cleveland, OH

Suzanna Mendoza, MS, RD, CSR, LDN
Renal Dietitian, US Renal Care Oak Brook Dialysis
Downers Grove, IL

Sean Paladini, MS, RDN, CSR
Renal Dietitian, George E. Wahlen Medical Center
Salt Lake City, UT

Preface

The second edition of the *Academy of Nutrition and Dietetics Pocket Guide to Chronic Kidney Disease and the Nutrition Care Process* is an update of the original pocket guide published in 2014. This new edition expands upon the first to include the 2020 update of the Nutrition Care Process (NCP) and Nutrition Care Process Terminology (NCPT).

This pocket guide is designed to assist the registered dietitian nutritionist in applying NCPT and evidence-based guidelines to assess, diagnose, and manage the nutrition care of patients with chronic kidney disease, as well as those who are on renal replacement therapy and those who have received a kidney transplant. In addition to the 2020 NCPT, this edition incorporates the 2020 Kidney Disease Outcomes Quality Initiative (KDOQI) nutrition guidelines, revised Kidney Disease Improving Global Outcomes (KDIGO) practice guidelines, and information from the 6th edition of the National Kidney Foundation Council on Renal Nutrition *Pocket Guide to Nutrition Assessment of the Patient with Kidney Disease*.

We hope that you find the second edition of the *Academy of Nutrition and Dietetics Pocket Guide to Chronic Kidney Disease and the Nutrition Care Process* helpful in mastering the use of NCPT and applying evidence-based guidelines to the care of your patients with kidney disease.

Acknowledgments

We would like to acknowledge several individuals for their help in the development of this book. Without their support, publication of the second edition of the *Academy of Nutrition and Dietetics Pocket Guide to Chronic Kidney Disease and the Nutrition Care Process* would not have been possible. First, we would like to thank our previous coauthor of the pocket guide, Maureen P. McCarthy, MPH, RD (retired). Maureen was the inspiration and leader responsible for the success of the first edition. We are grateful to our families for their support and encouragement while we worked on this edition of the pocket guide. We would also like to thank the Academy of Nutrition and Dietetics Product Strategy and Development Team including Stacey Zettle, MS, RDN and Betsy Hornick, MS, RDN. Each provided invaluable support and encouragement from the beginning to the end of this project. Last, thank you to the reviewers who volunteered their time and expertise to provide feedback on this project. We hope this edition will continue to provide renal nutrition practitioners with relevant Nutrition Care Process Terminology and evidence-based guidance to better assess, diagnose, treat, monitor, and document patient care.

About the Authors

Jessie M. Pavlinac, MS, RDN-AP, CSR, LD, FNKF, FAND, is a registered and licensed dietitian/nutritionist and a board-certified specialist in renal nutrition with masters degrees in nutrition science and health care management, and over 40 years of experience in renal and transplant nutrition. Jessie is currently a clinical instructor at Oregon Health and Science University (OHSU). She retired as manager of clinical nutrition at OHSU in 2020 where she also practiced in the areas of renal and transplant nutrition. Jessie also works as an associate instructor at Clackamas Community College and an adjunct instructor at Rutgers University. She has served in national leadership roles within the Academy of Nutrition and Dietetics including past Academy President, Speaker of the House of Delegates, and Chair of the Nutrition Care Process and Research Outcomes Committee, and has served on the Accreditation Council for Education in Nutrition and Dietetics (ACEND), the Academy Nominating Committee, and numerous other committees.

Jessie has also served in many leadership roles within the National Kidney Foundation and was recently awarded Fellowship. She serves on several editorial boards including the *Journal of Renal Nutrition* and the Academy of Nutrition and Dietetics Nutrition Care Manual and eatrightPREP course. She has given numerous presentations and authored articles on reimbursement for nutrition services, quality management, ethics, renal and transplant nutrition, and clinical nutrition management.

Jessie was honored to be one of the 2010 Winter Olympic Torchbearers. She is a fellow of the Academy of Nutrition and Dietetics and the National Kidney Foundation.

Arianna Aoun, MS, RDN, LD, is a registered and licensed dietitian with 20 years of experience as a renal dietitian. Arianna is currently the dietetic internship director for the VA Northeast Ohio Healthcare System and adjunct faculty at Case Western Reserve University. Arianna served on the team that developed the Academy of Nutrition and Dietetics 2010 Evidence-Based Nutrition Practice Guidelines for Chronic Kidney Disease. She has also been involved in the development of the Department of Veterans Affairs/Department of Defense (VA/DoD) Clinical Practice Guidelines on the management of Chronic Kidney Disease and Overweight/Obesity.

Throughout her career Arianna has given multiple local, regional, and national presentations on renal nutrition and the nutrition care of bariatric surgery patients. Since 1999, she has volunteered with the Kidney Foundation of Ohio, Inc., serving on the Renal Symposium Development Committee and the Medical Advisory Board. Arianna was honored to be nominated and selected for the Ohio Outstanding Dietetic Educator Award in 2020. She enjoys spending time with her family and traveling.

Publisher's Note on Gender-Inclusive Language

The Academy of Nutrition and Dietetics encourages diversity and inclusion by striving to recognize, respect, and include differences in ability, age, creed, culture, ethnicity, gender, gender identity, political affiliation, race, religion, sexual orientation, size, and socioeconomic characteristics in the nutrition and dietetics profession.[1]

As part of our commitment to diversity and inclusion, all new and updated editions of professional books and practitioner resources published by the Academy of Nutrition and Dietetics will transition to the use of inclusive language. As appropriate, inclusive language, including person/persons, individual/individuals, or patient/patients, is used to respect and recognize transgender and nonbinary people. Where gender or sex is referred to in this book, it is important to note that gender was not further specified for study participants and specific recommendations for transgender people were not provided.

Existing guidelines for nutrition assessment and interventions rely primarily on gender-specific values and recommendations. As research continues to explore the unique health and nutrition needs of transgender people, nutrition and health practitioners can expand their knowledge and understanding by reviewing available resources that provide guidance for person-centered nutrition care of gender-diverse individuals.[2-4] The use of inclusive language is consistent with the American Medical Association's *AMA Manual of Style*[5] as well as other health professional groups and government organizations. The Academy of Nutrition and Dietetics will continue to evolve to adopt consensus best practices related to nutrition care of gender-diverse individuals that maximize inclusivity and improve equitable and evidence-based care.

1. IDEA Action Plan. Academy of Nutrition and Dietetics website. Accessed September 6, 2023. www.eatrightpro.org/-/media/images/eatrightpro-landing-pages/career-idea-plan.jpg
2. Rozga M, Linsenmeyer W, Cantwell Wood J, Darst V, Gradwell EK. Hormone therapy, health outcomes and the role of nutrition in transgender individuals: A scoping review. *Clinical Nutrition ESPEN*. 2020;40:42-56. doi:10.1016/j.clnesp.2020.08.011
3. Rahman R, Linsenmeyer WR. Caring for transgender patients and clients: nutrition-related clinical and psychosocial considerations. *J Acad Nutr Diet*. 2019;119(5):727-732. doi:10.1016/j.jand.2018.03.006CTICE
4. Fergusson P, Greenspan N, Maitland L, Huberdeau R. Towards providing culturally aware nutritional care for transgender people: key issues and considerations. *Can J Diet Pract Res*. 2018;79(2):74-79. doi:10.3148/cjdpr-2018-001
5. JAMA Network. *AMA Manual of Style*. 11th ed. Oxford University Press; 2020:543-544.

CHAPTER 1

Chronic Kidney Disease, Evidence-Based Practice, and the Nutrition Care Process

This guide incorporates nutrition care for chronic kidney disease (CKD) with the steps of the Nutrition Care Process (NCP)—nutrition assessment, nutrition diagnosis, nutrition intervention, and nutrition monitoring and evaluation—as outlined in the *Abridged Nutrition Care Process Terminology (NCPT) Reference Manual: Standardized Terminology for the Nutrition Care Process*[1] and the online electronic Nutrition Care Process Terminology (eNCPT)[2] published by the Academy of Nutrition and Dietetics. The following are also incorporated in the text, tables, and boxes in this guide:

- the Kidney Disease Outcomes Quality Initiative (KDOQI) clinical practice guideline for nutrition in CKD (2020 update),[3] which was developed by the Academy of Nutrition and Dietetics and the National Kidney Foundation (NKF)
- the Academy of Nutrition and Dietetics Evidence Analysis Library CKD practice guideline[4]
- recommendations from NKF-KDOQI publications on nutrition (2000)[5] and diabetes and CKD[6,7]

- diabetes management recommendations from Kidney Disease Improving Global Outcomes (KDIGO), an international consortium of professional and patient-based organizations dedicated to kidney disease[8]
- recommendations from collaborative publications by NKF-KDOQI and KDIGO, specifically the guidelines on kidney transplant,[9,10] CKD evaluation and management,[11,12] anemia in CKD,[13-16] blood pressure in CKD,[17-20] dyslipidemia management in CKD,[21-23] and CKD–mineral and bone disorder (CKD-MBD)[24-27]
- criteria for reimbursement and required documentation established by the US Centers for Medicare & Medicaid Services (CMS) Conditions for Coverage (CfC) for end-stage renal disease (ESRD) facilities and CMS Medicare Part B reimbursement criteria for medical nutrition therapy (MNT) for CKD and renal transplant[28-31]
- key points from the American Society for Parenteral and Enteral Nutrition (ASPEN) clinical guidelines regarding nutrition support for acute and chronic renal failure in adults and ASPEN critical care guidelines for renal failure in adults[32,33]

Findings and recommendations from these sources are integrated into the chapters to which they apply—Chapter 2: Nutrition Assessment, Chapter 3: Nutrition Diagnosis, Chapter 4: Nutrition Intervention Part 1—Planning the Nutrition Prescription, Chapter 5, Nutrition Intervention Part 2—Implementation, and Chapter 6: Nutrition Monitoring and Evaluation.

Medical Nutrition Therapy and the Nutrition Care Process in Chronic Kidney Disease

Stages of Chronic Kidney Disease

In 2002, NKF-KDOQI published a five-stage system for classifying CKD.[34] The *2012 KDIGO Clinical Practice Guidelines for the Evaluation and Management of CKD* maintained the glomerular filtration rate (GFR) ranges for CKD stages 1 through 5 but split stage 3 into two categories: 3a and 3b (see Table 1.1).[11]

TABLE 1.1 Stages of Chronic Kidney Disease[11]	
Stage	Glomerular filtration rate, mL/min/1.73 m²
1	≥90 with kidney damage
2	60-89
3a	45-59
3b	30-44
4	15-29
5 and 5D (D = dialysis)	<15

Patients who are post transplant have varying levels of renal function. Their CKD stage should be determined based on their estimated glomerular filtration rate (eGFR), with MNT applied accordingly. The NKF and the American Society of Nephrology (ASN) appointed a task force to evaluate eGFR calculation methods. The goal of the collaboration was to determine a method of calculating eGFR without using the race variable, which was noted to be a societal interpretation and had no biological impact or relevance.[35] In 2021, the NKF/ASN task force[35] released three recommendations:

1. Immediately implement the "Chronic Kidney Disease Epidemiology Collaboration (CKD-EPI) creatinine equation refit without the race variable in all laboratories."

2. Increase the use of cystatin C "to confirm estimated GFR in adults for clinical decision making."

3. Focus on "new endogenous filtration markers and interventions to eliminate racial and ethnic disparities."

Medical Nutrition Therapy and the Nutrition Care Process

MNT is an essential intervention to promote ideal health parameters. Patients with various health conditions and illnesses can improve their health and quality of life when learning to adhere to MNT recommendations. During MNT interventions, registered dietitian nutritionists (RDNs) educate and counsel patients on behavioral and lifestyle changes essential to encourage positive lifelong eating habits and health measures. MNT utilizes evidence-based nutrition to execute the steps of the NCP, as outlined in Box 1.1.[36]

> **BOX 1.1 Steps of the Nutrition Care Process[36]**
>
> The steps of the Nutrition Care Process follow the acronym **ADIME:**
> - Perform a comprehensive nutrition assessment (**A**) and reassessment
> - Determine the nutrition diagnosis (**D**)
> - Plan and implement a nutrition intervention (**I**) using evidence-based nutrition practice guidelines
> - Monitor (**M**) an individual's progress over subsequent visits with the registered dietitian nutritionist
> - Evaluate (**E**) an individual's progress over subsequent visits with the registered dietitian nutritionist

This pocket guide focuses on the appropriate MNT for CKD stages 1 through 5D, including post transplantation. Acute kidney injury is not addressed. Practitioners should individualize MNT; the focus will depend on the patient's stage of CKD, medical history, and whether the encounter is an initial or follow-up visit. For example, MNT provided for a patient with a history of CKD stage 5 and diabetes who has elevated potassium and phosphorus levels but hemoglobin A1c (HbA1c) of 6.8% would be different from MNT for a patient with CKD stage 3a and normal potassium and phosphorus levels but HbA1c of 9%. Nutrition prescriptions and interventions are discussed further in Chapters 4 and 5, respectively.

Reimbursement Overview

Medicare Part B reimburses MNT provided by an RDN or other qualified nutrition professional, with a physician referral, for patients whose GFR is between 15 and 59 mL/min/1.73 m² (predialysis).[29,37] Patients who are post–kidney transplant with any level of allograft function are covered by Medicare Part B for up to 3 years with a physician referral.[29] More information can be found on the CMS website (www.cms.gov; search for "MNT"). Table 1.2 provides a summary of Medicare Part B coverage for MNT for patients with CKD.[29,30,37]

TABLE 1.2 Medicare Part B Reimbursement for Medical Nutrition Therapy for Patients With Chronic Kidney Disease[29,30,37]

Timeline	Number of medical nutrition therapy units reimbursed[a]	Total hours per year
First year	12	3
Each subsequent year	8	2

[a] For patients with an estimated glomerular filtration rate of 15 to 59 mL/min/1.73 m² and patients who are post transplant.

Based on medical necessity, additional hours of MNT may be covered if the treating physician orders them because of a change in the patient's medical condition, diagnosis, or treatment regimen.[29,30] For the first 3 years after transplant, MNT is a Medicare Part B benefit regardless of GFR with a physician referral.[29] After that time period, however, only those posttransplant patients with continuing CKD and a physician referral are eligible for Medicare Part B reimbursement for MNT.[29]

Medicare Part B reimburses dialysis care when that care is delivered in a Medicare-approved outpatient dialysis facility, in the home, or via peritoneal dialysis (PD). A dietitian is required to "provide nutrition assessment, recommendations, counseling, and follow-up" to satisfy Medicare ESRD regulations.[38] Dialysis reimbursement is provided by the ESRD Prospective Payment System for up to three treatments per week, unless additional treatments are medically needed. All dialysis care, including renal MNT, is "bundled" into one payment per treatment.[38]

In 2021, the ESRD Treatment Choices model was introduced to promote patient selection of home dialysis and/or kidney transplant as a treatment modality and was rolled out in randomly selected geographic areas. With this new model, payment for MNT is rolled into payment for other dialysis care services.[38]

As a result of the COVID-19 pandemic, CMS expanded approval for telehealth visits.[39,40] With the end of the COVID-19 public health emergency, CMS has permanently authorized some types of telehealth care, but other telehealth flexibilities will expire December 31, 2024.[41]

Screening and Referral for Medical Nutrition Therapy Encounters

The 2010 Academy of Nutrition and Dietetics CKD guideline[4] and the 2020 KDOQI/Academy of Nutrition and Dietetics guideline[3] recommend the following practices for screening and referral of patients for care by an RDN or international equivalent:

- For adults with CKD stage 3 through 5D and post transplant, "it is reasonable to consider routine nutrition screening at least biannually with the intent of identifying those at risk of protein-energy wasting [PEW]."[3]
- MNT should be provided by the RDN for individuals with CKD because "MNT prevents and treats protein-energy malnutrition and mineral and electrolyte disorders and minimizes the impact of other comorbidities on the progression of kidney disease (eg, diabetes, obesity, hypertension, and disorders of lipid metabolism)."[4]
- MNT "should be initiated at diagnosis of CKD, in order to maintain adequate nutritional status, prevent disease progression, and delay renal replacement therapy (RRT) ... or transplant. MNT should be initiated at least 12 months prior to the anticipation of RRT."[4]

- For adults with CKD stage 3 through 5D and post transplant, "it is reasonable that a registered dietitian nutritionist (RDN) or an international equivalent conduct a comprehensive nutrition assessment (included but not limited to appetite, history of dietary intake, biochemical data, anthropometric measurements, and nutrition focused physical findings) at least within the first 90 days of starting dialysis, annually, or when indicated by nutrition screening or provider referral."[3]

The 2020 KDOQI/Academy of Nutrition and Dietetics work group[3] was not able to suggest one nutrition screening tool as performing better than others when evaluating patients with PEW.

The 2020 KDOQI/Academy of Nutrition and Dietetics guideline used the GRADE (Grading of Recommendations Assessment, Development and Evaluation) work group grading system to evaluate the evidence around the recommendations (see Box 1.2).[3,42] It is important to understand that not all recommendations are based on rigorous scientific evidence.

BOX 1.2 Strength of Recommendation and Quality of Evidence[3,42]

Strength of recommendation		Quality of evidence	
Level	Meaning	Grade	Meaning
1	"We recommend"	A	High quality
		B	Moderate quality
2	"We suggest"	C	Low quality
		D	Very low quality

In addition to evaluating the clinical evidence, the 2020 KDOQI/Academy of Nutrition and Dietetics work group also determined the strength of the recommendations. A strong recommendation received a level 1 ("we recommend") rating, meaning most individuals should receive the recommended course of action. A weak recommendation received a level 2 ("we suggest") rating, meaning that the action may be appropriate for some patients but the clinician should spend time helping patients make an individualized decision.[3] **As appropriate, the strength of the recommendations and the grade of evidence are included throughout this guide (with the number and letter noted in parentheses in the respective statement).**

Medical Nutrition Therapy Based on Chronic Kidney Disease Stage

The RDN evaluates the stage of CKD and prioritizes the strategy for MNT based on nutrition issues that arise during that stage. In addition, the RDN assesses the patient's level of interest in learning about the stage of CKD and the available social support and, on that basis, tailors MNT education and counseling. MNT for posttransplantation patients should be based on posttransplant renal function, which may decline over time.

Stage 3 and Post Transplantation

In clinical practice, evidence-based guidelines for MNT should be applied as appropriate based on a review of the patient's medical history (eg, diabetes, hypertension, lipid disorders, or obesity), stage of CKD (including kidney transplant), nutritional status, and any mineral or electrolyte imbalances. The RDN should plan to coordinate the care of the patient with CKD with the interdisciplinary team to maximize the individual's care.[3,4,28]

Stage 4 and Post Transplantation

Because CKD stage 4 is defined by an eGFR of 15 to 29 mL/min/1.73 m^2, MNT for CKD and posttransplant patients with this stage is covered by Medicare Part B.[11,29] As in earlier stages of CKD, MNT is based on a thorough assessment and includes coordination of care.

Stage 5 Not on Dialysis and Post Transplantation

CKD stage 5 not on dialysis is defined by an eGFR of less than 15 mL/min/1.73 m^2.[11] Medicare Part B provides MNT coverage only for patients with an eGFR of 15 mL/min/1.73 m² or greater within stage 5 CKD or for posttransplant patients with this level of renal function.[37] As in earlier stages of CKD, MNT is based on a thorough assessment and includes coordination of care.

Stage 5D Hemodialysis and Peritoneal Dialysis

CKD stage 5D is defined by the initiation of renal replacement therapy (either maintenance hemodialysis or PD).[17] Nutritional status should be evaluated using a combination of measures, such as protein and energy intake, body composition, and functional status.[3,5]

CMS has released CfC for ESRD, which outlines the mandatory nutrition care plan and documentation to be completed for each patient on dialysis.[28] Box 1.3 summarizes the CfC and corresponding interpretive guidelines that relate to the four steps of the NCP. Interpretive guidelines are published by government agencies such as the CMS to guide surveyors, who are applying standards such as the CfC in the field.[43-45]

BOX 1.3 Medicare Conditions for Coverage Mandates Related to the Nutrition Care Process and Documentation[43-45]

Nutrition assessment

Condition for Coverage (CfC) §494.80 describes requirements for patient assessment.

Interpretative Guideline (IG) Tags V500 to V515 describe information to be included in assessments.
- IG Tag V509 is specific to nutrition.
- Topics discussed in other tags, such as factors associated with renal bone disease, also relate to nutrition and may be completely or partially addressed by the nephrology registered dietitian nutritionist (RDN) in accordance with accepted practice patterns at a given end-stage renal disease facility.

Nutrition diagnosis

Nutrition diagnosis is not mandated by the US Centers for Medicare & Medicaid Services but is a vital component of what the RDN does.

The nutrition diagnosis should be included in documentation of nutrition care.

Continued on next page

> **BOX 1.3 Medicare Conditions for Coverage Mandates Related to the Nutrition Care Process and Documentation (cont.)**[43-45]
>
> ***Nutrition intervention (including care plan) and nutrition monitoring and evaluation***
>
> CfC § 494.90 states that an interdisciplinary team must develop and implement a comprehensive plan of care (POC) that describes services needed (ie, interventions) and outcomes (ie, monitoring and evaluation step of the Nutrition Care Process).
>
> IG Tag 545 sets expectations for an outcome-oriented POC related to nutritional status.

References

1. Academy of Nutrition and Dietetics. *Abridged Nutrition Care Process Terminology (NCPT) Reference Manual: Standardized Terminology for the Nutrition Care Process*. Academy of Nutrition and Dietetics; 2018.
2. Academy of Nutrition and Dietetics. Electronic Nutrition Care Process Terminology (eNCPT). Accessed November 29, 2022. www.ncpro.org
3. Ikizler TA, Burrowes JD, Byham-Gray LD, et al. KDOQI clinical practice guideline for nutrition in CKD: 2020 update. *J Kidney Dis*. 2020; 76(3 suppl 1):S1-S107. doi:10.1053/j.ajkd.2020.05.006
4. Academy of Nutrition and Dietetics Evidence Analysis Library. Chronic kidney disease (CKD) guideline. 2010. Accessed August 11, 2022. www.andeal.org/topic.cfm?cat=3927&highlight=kidney&home=1
5. Kidney Disease Outcomes Quality Initiative, National Kidney Foundation. Clinical practice guidelines for nutrition in chronic renal failure. *Am J Kidney Dis*. 2000;35(6 suppl 2):S17-S104. doi:10.1053/ajkd.2000.v35.aajkd03517
6. Kidney Disease Outcomes Quality Initiative. KDOQI clinical practice guidelines and clinical practice recommendations for diabetes and chronic kidney disease. *Am J Kidney Dis*. 2007;49(2 suppl 2):S12-S154. doi:10.1053/j.ajkd.2006.12.005
7. National Kidney Foundation. KDOQI clinical practice guideline for diabetes and CKD: 2012 update. *Am J Kidney Dis*. 2012;60(5):850-886. doi:10.1053/j.ajkd.2012.07.005

8. Kidney Disease Improving Global Outcomes. KDIGO clinical practice guideline for diabetes management in chronic kidney disease. *Kidney Int Suppl.* 2020;98(4S):S1-S115.
9. Kidney Disease Improving Global Outcomes (KDIGO) Transplant Work Group. KDIGO clinical practice guideline for the care of kidney transplant recipients. *Am J Transplant.* 2009;9(suppl 3):S1-S155. doi:10.1111/j.1600-6143.2009.02834.x
10. Bia M, Adey DB, Bloom RD, Chan L, Kulkarni S, Tomlanovich S. KDOQI US commentary on the 2009 KDIGO clinical practice guideline for the care of kidney transplant recipients. *Am J Kidney Dis.* 2010;56(2):189-218. doi:10.1053/j.ajkd.2010.04.010
11. Kidney Disease Improving Global Outcomes. KDIGO 2012 clinical practice guideline for the evaluation and management of chronic kidney disease. *Kidney Int Suppl.* 2013;3(1):26-32. https://kdigo.org/wp-content/uploads/2017/02/KDIGO_2012_CKD_GL.pdf
12. Inker LA, Astor BC, Fox CH, et al. KDOQI US commentary on the 2012 KDIGO clinical practice guideline for the evaluation and management of CKD. *Am J Kidney Dis.* 2014;63(5):713-735. doi:10.1053/j.ajkd.2014.01.416
13. Kidney Disease Outcomes Quality Initiative, National Kidney Foundation. KDOQI clinical practice guidelines and clinical practice recommendations for anemia in chronic kidney disease. *Am J Kidney Dis.* 2006;47(5 suppl 3):S11-S145. doi:10.1053/j.ajkd.2006.03.010
14. Kidney Disease Outcomes Quality Initiative. KDOQI clinical practice guideline and clinical practice recommendations for anemia in chronic kidney disease: 2007 update of hemoglobin target. *Am J Kidney Dis.* 2007;50(3):471-530. doi:10.1053/j.ajkd.2007.06.008
15. Kidney Disease Improving Global Outcomes. KDIGO clinical practice guideline for anemia in chronic kidney disease. *Kidney Int Suppl.* 2012;2(4):279-335. https://kdigo.org/wp-content/uploads/2016/10/KDIGO-2012-Anemia-Guideline-English.pdf
16. Kliger AS, Foley RN, Goldfarb DS, et al. KDOQI US commentary on the 2012 KDIGO clinical practice guideline for anemia in CKD. *Am J Kidney Dis.* 2013;62(5):849-859. doi:10.1053/j.ajkd.2013.06.008
17. Kidney Disease Outcomes Quality Initiative (K/DOQI). K/DOQI clinical practice guidelines on hypertension and antihypertensive agents in chronic kidney disease. *Am J Kidney Dis.* 2004;43(5 suppl 1):S1-S290.
18. Kidney Disease Improving Global Outcomes. KDIGO clinical practice guideline for the management of blood pressure in chronic kidney disease. *Kidney Int Suppl.* 2012;2(5):v-414. https://kdigo.org/wp-content/uploads/2016/10/KDIGO-2012-Blood-Pressure-Guideline-English.pdf

19. Taler SJ, Agarwal R, Bakris GL, et al. KDOQI US commentary on the 2012 KDIGO clinical practice guideline for management of blood pressure in CKD. *Am J Kidney Dis*. 2013;62(2):201-213. doi:10.1053/j.ajkd.2013.03.018

20. Kidney Disease Improving Global Outcomes (KDIGO) Blood Pressure Work Group. KDIGO 2021 clinical practice guideline for the management of blood pressure in chronic kidney disease. *Kidney Int*. 2021;99(3 suppl):S1-S87. doi:10.1016/j.kint.2020.11.003

21. Kidney Disease Outcomes Quality Initiative (K/DOQI) Group. K/DOQI clinical practice guidelines for management of dyslipidemias in patients with kidney disease. *Am J Kidney Dis*. 2003;41(4 suppl 3):I-S91.

22. Kidney Disease Improving Global Outcomes. KDIGO clinical practice guidelines for lipid management in chronic kidney disease. *Kidney Int Suppl*. 2013;3(3):259-305. https://kdigo.org/wp-content/uploads/2017/02/KDIGO-2013-Lipids-Guideline-English.pdf

23. Sarnak MJ, Bloom R, Muntner P, et al. KDOQI US commentary on the 2013 KDIGO clinical practice guideline for lipid management in CKD. *Am J Kidney Dis*. 2015;65(3):354-366. doi:10.1053/j.ajkd.2014.10.005

24. Kidney Disease Improving Global Outcomes (KDIGO) CKD-MBD Work Group. KDIGO clinical practice guideline for the diagnosis, evaluation, prevention, and treatment of chronic kidney disease–mineral and bone disorder (CKD-MBD). *Kidney Int Suppl*. 2009;(113):S1-S130. doi:10.1038/ki.2009.188

25. Uhlig K, Berns JS, Kestenbaum B, et al. KDOQI US commentary on the 2009 KDIGO clinical practice guideline for the diagnosis, evaluation, and treatment of CKD–mineral and bone disorder (CKD-MBD). *Am J Kidney Dis*. 2010;55(5):773-799. doi:10.1053/j.ajkd.2010.02.340

26. Kidney Disease Improving Global Outcomes (KDIGO) CKD-MBD Update Work Group. KDIGO 2017 clinical practice guideline update for the diagnosis, evaluation, prevention, and treatment of chronic kidney disease–mineral and bone disorder (CKD-MBD). *Kidney Int Suppl*. 2017;7(1):1-59. doi:10.1016/j.kisu.2017.04.001

27. Isakova T, Nickolas TL, Denburg M, et al. KDOQI US commentary on the 2017 KDIGO clinical practice guideline update for the diagnosis, evaluation, prevention, and treatment of chronic kidney disease–mineral and bone disorder (CKD-MBD). *Am J Kidney Dis*. 2017;70(6):737-751. doi:10.1053/j.ajkd.2017.07.019

28. US Centers for Medicare and Medicaid Services. Conditions for Coverage for end-stage renal disease facilities. *Fed Regist*. 2008;73(73):20370-20484. www.cms.gov/Regulations-and-Guidance/Legislation/CFCsAndCoPs/Downloads/ESRDfinalrule0415.pdf

29. US Centers for Medicare and Medicaid Services. Coverage information. In: *The Guide to Medicare Preventive Services*. 4th ed. US Department of Health and Human Services; 2011:126-128. Accessed February 8, 2023. www.curemd.com/the_guide.pdf

30. Academy of Nutrition and Dietetics. General comparisons of DSMT benefits and MNT Medicare benefits. eatrightPRO website. Accessed August 9, 2020. www.eatrightpro.org/payment/medicare/providing-service-and-billing/general-comparisons-of-dsmt-benefits-and-mnt-medicare-benefits

31. US Centers for Medicare and Medicaid Services. Quality, safety and oversight-guidance to laws and regulations: dialysis. CMS.gov website. Modified January 25, 2022. Accessed August 11, 2022. www.cms.gov/Medicare/Provider-Enrollment-and-Certification/GuidanceforLawsAndRegulations/Dialysis.html

32. Brown RO, Compher C; American Society for Parenteral and Enteral Nutrition Board of Directors. A.S.P.E.N. clinical guidelines: nutrition support in adult acute and chronic renal failure. *JPEN J Parenter Enteral Nutr.* 2010;34(4):366-377. doi:10.1177/0148607110374577

33. McClave SA, Taylor BE, Martindale RG, et al. Guidelines for the provision and assessment of nutrition support therapy in the adult critically ill patient: Society of Critical Care Medicine (SCCM) and American Society for Parenteral and Enteral Nutrition (A.S.P.E.N.) *JPEN J Parenter Enteral Nutr.* 2016;40(2):159-211. doi:10.1177/0148607115621863

34. National Kidney Foundation. K/DOQI clinical practice guidelines for chronic kidney disease: evaluation, classification, and stratification. *Am J Kidney Dis.* 2002;39(2 suppl 1):S1-S266.

35. Delgado C, Baweja M, Crews DC, et al. A unifying approach for GFR estimation: recommendations of the NKF-ASN Task Force on Reassessing the Inclusion of Race in Diagnosing Kidney Disease. *Am J Kidney Dis.* 2022;79(2):268-288. doi:10.1053/j.ajkd.2021.08.003

36. Academy of Nutrition and Dietetics. Nutrition Care Process. Accessed November 5, 2021. www.ncpro.org/nutrition-care-process

37. Centers for Medicare & Medicaid Services. Pub 100-04 Medicare Claims Processing. May 20, 2022. Accessed August 30, 2023. www.cms.gov/files/document/r11426cp.pdf

38. Academy of Nutrition and Dietetics. ESRD services (outpatient dialysis). Accessed July 11, 2022. eatrightPRO website. www.eatrightpro.org/payment/coding-and-billing/places-of-service-and-specific-health-care-services/esrd-services

39. US Centers for Medicare and Medicaid Services. MLN Fact Sheet: Telehealth Services. June 2021. Accessed August 11, 2022. www.cms.gov/Outreach-and-Education/Medicare-Learning-Network-MLN/MLNProducts/downloads/telehealthsrvcsfctsht.pdf

40. US Centers for Medicare and Medicaid Services. Medicare Telemedicine Health Care Provider Fact Sheet. March 17, 2020. Accessed August 11, 2022. www.cms.gov/newsroom/fact-sheets/medicare-telemedicine-health-care-provider-fact-sheet
41. Health Resources and Services Administration. Telehealth policy changes after the COVID-19 public health emergency. Telehealth. HHS.gov website. Accessed July 28, 2023. https://telehealth.hhs.gov/providers/telehealth-policy/policy-changes-after-the-covid-19-public-health-emergency
42. Schunemann H, Brozek J, Guyatt G, Oxman A, eds.; GRADE Workgroup. *GRADE Handbook for Grading Quality of Evidence and Strength of Recommendations*. 2013. Accessed July 23, 2022. https://gdt.gradepro.org/app/handbook/handbook.html#h.trgki08omk7z
43. US Centers for Medicare and Medicaid Services. Quality, safety and oversight: guidance to laws and regulations—dialysis. ESRD program interpretive guidance. CMS.gov website. Accessed July 23, 2022. www.cms.gov/Medicare/Provider-Enrollment-and-Certification/GuidanceforLawsAndRegulations/Dialysis
44. US Centers for Medicare and Medicaid Services. ESRD surveyor training interpreter guidance. Final version 1.1. October 3, 2008. Accessed August 11, 2022. www.cms.gov/Medicare/Provider-Enrollment-and-Certification/GuidanceforLawsAndRegulations/Downloads/esrdpgmguidance.pdf
45. McCarthy M, Asbell D. A Renal Nutrition Forum series with practice-based examples of the Nutrition Care Process (NCP): where does nutrition diagnosis fit in the new Conditions for Coverage? *Renal Nutr Forum*. 2009;28(2):20-23.

CHAPTER 2

Nutrition Assessment

Throughout the remaining chapters of this guide, a case study approach will be used to illustrate the management of chronic kidney disease (CKD). The case study is presented in installments at the end of each chapter, adding details pertinent to the Nutrition Care Process (NCP) step discussed in that chapter.

The process of *nutrition assessment* includes obtaining, verifying, and interpreting data to identify a nutrition problem or diagnosis. Nutrition assessment is ongoing and involves comparing the patient's data parameters to standards or expected values for the overall condition.[1,2] Nutrition assessment for patients with CKD requires an understanding of kidney physiology, the nutritional ramifications in the various stages of CKD, and how medical management (including medications) affects the nutritional status of the patient. This chapter discusses the five domains of nutrition assessment as they relate to patients with CKD:

- food/nutrition-related history
- anthropometric measurements
- biochemical data, medical tests, and procedures
- nutrition focused physical findings
- patient history

The terminology used is from the *Abridged Nutrition Care Process Terminology (NCPT) Reference Manual: Standardized Terminology for the Nutrition Care Process*[1] and the eNCPT online manual (www.ncpro.org).[2] Comparative standards for CKD for energy, micronutrients, macronutrients, fluid needs, and weight recommendations are included in this guide.[1,2]

Food/Nutrition-Related History

The food/nutrition related data needed to perform an assessment of a patient with CKD are discussed in detail in the Box 2.1.[2]

> **BOX 2.1 Food/Nutrition Related Data Needed to Perform an Assessment[2]**
>
> ### Food and nutrient intake
>
> Energy intake
>
> Food and beverage intake
>
> Enteral and parenteral intake
>
> Bioactive substance intake
> - Alcohol
> - Bioactive substance
> - Caffeine
>
> Macronutrient intake
> - Fat
> - Cholesterol
> - Protein
> - Amino acid
> - Carbohydrate
> - Fiber
>
> Micronutrient intake
> - Vitamin
> - Mineral/element
>
> Food and nutrition component intake
> - Consistency modifier
>
> ### Food and nutrient administration
>
> Diet history
> - Diet order
> - Diet experience
> - Eating environment
> - Enteral and parenteral nutrition administration
> - Fasting

BOX 2.1 Food/Nutrition Related Data Needed to Perform an Assessment[2] (cont.)

Medication and complementary/alternative medicine use
Medications
Complementary/alternative medicine

Knowledge, beliefs, and attitudes
Food and nutrition knowledge
Food and nutrition skill
Beliefs and attitudes

Behavior
Adherence
Avoidance behavior
Bingeing and purging behavior
Mealtime behavior
Social network

Factors affecting access to food and food/nutrition related supplies
Food and nutrition program participation
Safe food availability
Safe water availability
Food- and nutrition-related supplies availability
Food and nutrition sanitation

Physical activity and function
Breastfeeding assessment
Nutrition-related activities of daily living and instrumental activities of daily living
Physical activity
Factors affecting access to physical activity

Nutrition related, patient-centered measures
Nutrition quality of life
Body composition, growth, and/or weight history
Acid-base balance

Continued on next page

> **BOX 2.1 Food/Nutrition Related Data Needed to Perform an Assessment[2] (cont.)**
>
> ***Nutrition related, patient-centered measures (continued)***
> Electrolyte and renal profile
> Essential fatty acid profile
> Gastrointestinal profile
> Glucose/endocrine profile
> Inflammatory profile
> Lipid profile
> Metabolic rate profile
> Mineral profile
> Nutritional anemia profile
> Protein profile
> Urine profile
> Vitamin profile

Gathering information on the following will serve as the basis for developing a CKD-appropriate nutrition prescription and education plan:

- the current nutrition prescription or pattern the patient follows;
- previous nutrition counseling/education;
- beliefs and attitudes around food; and
- food and nutrition knowledge regarding the protein, sodium, potassium, and phosphorus content of foods.

The availability of food, the ability to prepare foods, and the eligibility or need for food and nutrition assistance programs will also influence the care plan. The nutrition prescription must be developed based on the CKD stage and other comorbid conditions, if any. Specific guidelines for the nutrition prescription are described in Chapter 4.

Medication history and current medication usage, including complementary/alternative therapies, significantly affect the nutrition assessment and nutrition prescription of the patient with CKD. Common classes of medications used with these patients include antihypertensive, phosphate-binding, hypoglycemic, and cardiac agents. Assessment of medications and supplements should include their phosphorus and potassium content (particularly of over-the-counter products and dietary supplements); effect of the medication(s) on the kidneys with regard to sodium, potassium, and fluid elimination; composition of the phosphate binders; and impact of the medications on bone health and soft tissue calcification. Boxes 2.2 through 2.6 provide information about common medications used by individuals with CKD.[3-13]

BOX 2.2 Antihypertensive Medications Used in Chronic Kidney Disease[3,4]

	Examples	Chronic kidney disease–relevant adverse effect
Thiazides	chlorothiazide (Diuril)	Decreased serum potassium
	hydrochlorothiazide (Microzide, HydroDiuril)	
	indapamide (Lozol)	
	metolazone (Mykrox, Zaroxolyn)	
	polythiazide (Renese)	
Loop diuretics	bumetanide (Bumex)	Decreased serum potassium
	furosemide (Lasix)	
	torsemide (Dyrenium)	
Potassium-sparing medications	amiloride (Midamor)	Increased serum potassium
	triamterene (Dyrenium)	
	spironolactone (Aldactone, CaroSpir)	
Aldosterone receptor blockers	eplerenone (Inspra)	Increased serum potassium
	spironolactone (Aldactone)	

Continued on next page

BOX 2.2 Antihypertensive Medications Used in Chronic Kidney Disease (cont.)[3,4]

	Examples	Chronic kidney disease–relevant adverse effect
Beta blockers	atenolol (Tenormin)	Constipation, nausea, edema
	betaxolol (Kerlone)	
	bisoprolol (Zebeta)	
	metoprolol (Lopressor)	
	extended-release metoprolol (Toprol XL)	
	nadolol (Corgard)	
	propranolol (Inderal)	
	long-acting propranolol (Inderal LA)	
	timolol (Blocadren)	
Beta blockers with intrinsic sympathomimetic activity	acebutolol (Sectral)	Diarrhea
	penbutolol (Levatol)	
Combined alpha and beta blockers	carvedilol (Coreg)	Published data not available
	labetalol (Normodyne, Trandate)	
Angiotensin-converting enzyme inhibitors	benazepril (Lotensin)	Increased serum potassium, metallic or salty taste
	catopril (Capoten)	
	enalapril (Vasotec)	
	fosinopril (Monopril)	
	lisinopril (Prinivil, Zestril)	
	moexipril (Univasc)	
	perindopril (Aceon)	
	quinapril (Accupril)	
	ramipril (Altace)	
	trandolapril (Mavik)	

BOX 2.2 Antihypertensive Medications Used in Chronic Kidney Disease (cont.)[3,4]

	Examples	Chronic kidney disease–relevant adverse effect
Angiotensin II receptor blockers/ antagonists	candesartan (Atacand) eprosartan (Teveten) irbesartan (Avapro) losartan (Cozaar) olmesartan (Benicar) telmisartan (Micardis) valsartan (Diovan)	Increased serum potassium, salty or metallic taste, nausea, diarrhea, dyspepsia
Calcium channel blockers		
Nondihydropyridines	extended-release diltiazem (Cardizem CD, Dilacor XR, Tiazac, and Cardizem LA) immediate-release verapamil (Calan, Isoptin) long-acting verapamil (Calan SR, Isoptin SR) extended-release verapamil hydrochloride (Covera HS, Verelan PM)	Constipation, nausea, edema
Dihydropyridines	amlodipine (Norvasc) felodipine (Plendil) isradipine (Dynacirc CR) long-acting nifedipine (Adalat CC, Procardia XL) nisoldipine (Sular)	Constipation, nausea, edema

Continued on next page

BOX 2.2 Antihypertensive Medications Used in Chronic Kidney Disease (cont.)[3,4]

	Examples	Chronic kidney disease–relevant adverse effect
Alpha-1 blockers	doxazosin (Cardura) prazosin (Minipress) terazosin (Hytrin)	Edema
Central alpha-2 agonists and other centrally acting drugs	clonidine (Catapres) clonidine patch (Catapres-TTS) methyldopa (Aldomet) reserpine (Serpasil), guanfacine (Intuniv/Tenex)	Dry mouth, nausea, vomiting, constipation, weight gain
Direct vasodilators	hydralazine (Apresoline) minoxidil (Loniten)	Edema

BOX 2.3 Phosphate-Binding Medications Used in Chronic Kidney Disease[3,5-7]

Aluminum hydroxide

Forms:	Liquid, tablet, capsule
Mineral content:	25 to 525 mg aluminum per tablet
Estimated potential binding capacity:	22.3 mg phosphate (PO_4) bound per 5 mL 14.3 mg PO_4 bound per tablet
Potential advantages:	Effective phosphate binder
Potential disadvantages:	Aluminum toxicity; altered bone mineral integrity; dementia

(Note: Aluminum hydroxide is not recommended except for a very brief period secondary to danger of aluminum accumulation.)

Example:	Amphojel

BOX 2.3 Phosphate-Binding Medications Used in Chronic Kidney Disease (cont.)[3,5-7]

Calcium acetate

Forms:	Capsule, tablet
Mineral content:	25% elemental calcium (250 mg calcium per gram)
Estimated potential binding capacity:	45 mg PO_4 bound per gram
Potential advantages:	Effective binder; less calcium load than calcium carbonate with same binding capacity
Potential disadvantages:	Increased potential for hypercalcemia and parathyroid hormone (PTH) suppression; gastrointestinal (GI) symptoms; large pill size
Example:	PhosLo, Calphron, Eliphos, Phoslyra

Calcium carbonate

Forms:	Liquid, tablet, chewable, capsule, gum
Mineral content:	40% elemental calcium (400 mg calcium per gram)
Estimated potential binding capacity:	39 mg of PO_4 bound per gram
Potential advantages:	Effective; inexpensive; can be used as a calcium supplement
Potential disadvantages:	Increased calcium load with potential for hypercalcemia and PTH suppression; GI symptoms
Example:	TUMS

Continued on next page

BOX 2.3 Phosphate-Binding Medications Used in Chronic Kidney Disease (cont.)[3,5-7]

Calcium citrate

Forms:	Capsule, tablet
Mineral content:	22% elemental calcium
Estimated potential binding capacity:	Published data not available.
Potential advantages:	None
Potential disadvantages:	Not recommended; citrate enhances aluminum absorption and causes GI symptoms
Example:	Citracal

Ferric citrate

Forms:	Tablet
Mineral content:	Iron
Estimated potential binding capacity:	19.1 to 19.8 mg phosphorus per gram of ferric citrate
Potential advantages:	Improves ferritin and transferrin saturation levels and reduces intravenous iron and erythropoiesis-stimulating agent requirements
Potential disadvantages:	Do not use in hemochromatosis; can cause diarrhea or constipation
Example:	Auryxia

Lanthanum carbonate

Forms:	Tablet, chewable
Mineral content:	250 or 500 mg elemental lanthanum
Estimated potential binding capacity:	Published data not available.

BOX 2.3 Phosphate-Binding Medications Used in Chronic Kidney Disease (cont.)[3,5-7]

Lanthanum carbonate (continued)

Potential advantages:	Effective; lower pill burden with higher dosing (1,000 mg)
Potential disadvantages:	GI symptoms; cost; potential lanthanum accumulation
Example:	Fosrenol

Magnesium carbonate

Forms:	Capsule, tablet, liquid
Mineral content:	28% magnesium
Estimated potential binding capacity:	Published data not available.
Potential advantages:	Effective; potential for lower calcium load
Potential disadvantages:	GI symptoms; cost; potential for hypermagnesemia
Example:	Magonate, Magnebind

Sevelamer carbonate

Forms:	Tablet, powder
Mineral content:	None (does not contain calcium)
Estimated potential binding capacity:	Published data not available.
Potential advantages:	Effective; not absorbed; potential to improve bicarbonate levels and decrease low-density lipoprotein cholesterol (LDL-C) levels
Potential disadvantages:	GI symptoms; large pill size
	Avoid with history of severe constipation or bowel obstruction.
Example:	Renvela

Continued on next page

BOX 2.3 Phosphate-Binding Medications Used in Chronic Kidney Disease (cont.)[3,5-7]

Sevelamer hydrochloride

Forms:	Tablet
Mineral content:	None (does not contain calcium)
Estimated potential binding capacity:	Published data not available.
Potential advantages:	Effective; potential to lower LDL-C levels; smaller tablet available for those with difficulty swallowing
Potential disadvantages:	GI symptoms; potential for decreased bicarbonate levels; cost; large size of 800-mg tablet
Example:	Renagel

Sucroferric oxyhydroxide

Forms:	Chewable tablet. Do not swallow whole.
Mineral content:	Iron
	Each tablet contains 500 mg iron, but it is not absorbed.
Estimated potential binding capacity:	96% of available phosphate is bound when gastric pH is 2.5.
Potential advantages:	Effective; chewable tablet; reduced pill burden
Potential disadvantages:	Can cause diarrhea, dark-colored (black) stool, and stained teeth.
	Possible contraindicators include hemochromatosis, liver disease, stomach or intestinal disorder, or gastric or intestinal surgery.
Example:	Velphoro

BOX 2.4 Hypoglycemic Agents Used in Chronic Kidney Disease[8,9]

	Dosing for chronic kidney disease (CKD) stage 3 or 4 or stage 5 nondialysis/ kidney transplant	*Dosing for dialysis*
Insulin	Increased risk of hypoglycemia due to decreased clearance of insulin by the kidney; adjust dose based on patient's response.	Adjust dose based on patient's response.
First-generation sulfonylureas		
Acetohexamide, Tolazamide, and Tolbutamide	Avoid	Avoid
Chlorpropamide	Reduce dose by 50% when the glomerular filtration rate (GFR) is between 30 and 50 mL/min/1.73 m².	Avoid
Second-generation sulfonylureas		
Glipizide and Gliclazide	No dose adjustment needed.	No dose adjustment needed.
Glyburide and Glimepiride	Avoid	Avoid
Alpha-glucosidase inhibitors		
Acarbose and Miglitol	Not recommended if GFR is less than 25 mL/min/1.73 m².	Avoid
Biguanides		
Metformin	eGFR at or below 30 mL/min/1.73 m²	Reassess

BOX 2.4 Hypoglycemic Agents Used in Chronic Kidney Disease (cont.)[8,9]

	Dosing for CKD stage 3 or 4 or stage 5 nondialysis/ kidney transplant	Dosing for dialysis
Meglitinides		
Repaglinide	No dose adjustment needed.	No dose adjustment needed.
Nateglinide	Initiate at a low dose before meals.	Avoid
Thiazolidinediones		
Pioglitazone Rosiglitazone	No dose adjustment needed.	No dose adjustment needed.
Incretin mimetics		
Exenatide	No dose adjustment needed.	No dose adjustment needed.
Amylin analogs		
Pramlintide	No dose adjustment needed for GFR of 20 to 50 mL/min/1.73 m².	No data are available.
Dipeptidyl peptidase-4 inhibitors		
Sitagliptin	Reduce dose by 50% with GFR less than 45 mL/min/1.73 m² and by 75% when GFR is less than 30 mL/min/1.73 m².	Reduce dose by 75%.
Glucagon-like peptide-1 receptor agonists		
Dulaglutide Exenatide Exenatide extended release Semaglutide Liraglutide Lixisenatide	Not recommended with a GFR of less than 30 mL/min/1.73 m².	

BOX 2.4 Hypoglycemic Agents Used in Chronic Kidney Disease (cont.)[8,9]

| **Sodium-glucose cotransporter 2 inhibitors** | It is reasonable to withhold during times of prolonged fasting, surgery, or critical medical illness. | If a patient is at risk for hypovolemia, consider decreasing thiazide or loop diuretic dosages. |

BOX 2.5 Dosing Adjustments for Medicines Used to Treat Lipid Disorders in Chronic Kidney Disease[10-12]

Bile acid sequestrants

| Cholestyramine, colestipol, and colesevelam | No dose adjustment needed. |

Statins

Atorvastatin	No dose adjustment needed.
Fluvastatin and lovastatin	Use caution with late-stage chronic kidney disease (CKD). If glomerular filtration rate (GFR) is less than 30 mL/min/1.73 m^2, use caution with dosages greater than 20 mg/d.
Pravastatin	No dose adjustment needed.
Rosuvastatin	No dose adjustment needed with mild to moderate kidney disease. If GFR is less than 30 mL/min/1.73 m^2, do not exceed 10 mg/d.
Simvastatin	Initiate therapy at 5 mg/d in patients with severe kidney disease. Avoid use with cyclosporine.

Fibric acid derivatives

Gemfibrozil	Decrease dose or consider alternative therapy if creatinine is greater than 2 mg/dL.
Fenofibrate	Reduce dose by 50% in patients with GFR 60 to 90 mL/min/1.73 m^2.

Other

| Niacin and ezetimibe | No dose adjustments needed. |

BOX 2.6 Possible Effects of Selected Drugs on Nutrient Absorption and Utilization[3,13]

Alcohol	Increased excretion of magnesium, potassium, and zinc; impaired utilization of folic acid
Antacids	Decreased absorption of phosphorus and iron; bicarbonate decreases folate and iron absorption
Antibiotics	
Cycloserine	Decreased levels of vitamin B12, vitamin B6, and folate
Neomycin	Decreased absorption of fat, lactose, protein, vitamins (A, D, K, and B12), calcium, potassium, and iron
Isoniazid	Pyridoxine (vitamin B6) deficiency
Tetracycline	Binds with calcium, magnesium, iron, and zinc
Tobramycin	Increased urinary loss of potassium and magnesium
Anticoagulants	Decreased vitamin K–dependent coagulation factors
Anticonvulsants	Increased need for vitamins (K, D, and B12), folic acid, calcium, and magnesium; pyridoxine may increase drug effect
Antigout	Increased excretion of potassium, sodium, calcium, magnesium, amino acids, chloride, and riboflavin (vitamin B2)
Antiproliferative (*azathioprine; mycophenolate*)	Nausea, vomiting, mucositis, altered taste, folate deficiency, and increased nutrient needs with infection; possible bone marrow suppression in combination with antigout medications

BOX 2.6 Possible Effects of Selected Drugs on Nutrient Absorption and Utilization (cont.) [3,13]

Calcineurin inhibitors

Cyclosporine A	Increased serum potassium and glucose as well as hyperglycemia and hyperlipidemia
Tacrolimus	Increased potassium and sodium retention, increased loss of magnesium, and hyperglycemia

Corticosteroids — Hyperglycemia; increased protein catabolism or decreased protein synthesis; decreased absorption of calcium, phosphorus, and potassium; increased needs for vitamin B6, folate, vitamins C and D, and zinc; impaired wound healing

Diuretics — Increased urinary excretion of magnesium, zinc, potassium, thiamin (vitamin B1)

Note: Spironolactone (acts in distal renal tubule) is potassium sparing.

Hypocholesterolemics — Decreased absorption of fat, carotene, vitamins (A, D, K, and B12), and iron

Laxatives — Increased fecal loss of fat, calcium, potassium, magnesium, fluids, most vitamins, and carotene

Mineral oil — Decreased absorption of vitamins (A, D, and E), potassium, and calcium; effects may not be clinically significant

Anthropometric Measurements

Body composition, growth, and weight history are needed to perform a nutrition assessment of a patient with CKD.[1,2] The 2020 Kidney Disease Outcomes Quality Initiative (KDOQI)/Academy of Nutrition and Dietetics guideline[14] includes the following statement concerning assessment of body weight for adults with CKD stage 3 through 5D or post transplantation:

*It is reasonable that a registered dietitian nutritionist (RDN) or an international equivalent conduct a comprehensive nutrition assessment (including but not limited to appetite, history of dietary intake, body weight and body mass index, biochemical data, anthropometric measurements, and nutrition focused physical findings) at least within the first 90 days of starting dialysis, annually, or when indicated by nutrition screening or provider referral **(OPINION)**.*

The Academy of Nutrition and Dietetics[15] systematic review of the literature on anthropometric assessment in patients with CKD stage 1 through 5 (nondialysis) identified the following recommendations:

- Use clinical judgment in assessing body weight. There is a lack of standard reference norms for this population; therefore, clinical judgment must be used when determining which weight to use in assessment—that is, actual measured weight, history of weight changes, serial weight measurements, or weight adjusted for edema.
- Use published weight norms with caution. Ideal body weight, the Hamwi method to determine optimal body weight, standard body weight, BMI, and adjusted body weight all have drawbacks in the assessment of body weight in patients with CKD.
- In the assessment of body composition, consider that patients with CKD have altered body composition compared to healthy individuals.

- In body composition assessment, use valid measurements and methodology such as anthropometrics (including waist circumference and BMI) and body compartment estimates; there are no reference standards for assessing body composition in this population.

Obesity is common in patients with CKD. Box 2.7[16] lists the BMI classification system for obesity, and Box 2.8 on page 34 presents proposed mechanisms for the association of obesity with CKD.

BOX 2.7 International Classification of Adult Weight According to BMI[16]

Classification	Principal BMI cutoff point[a]
Severe thinness	Less than 16
Moderate thinness	16 through 16.99
Mild thinness	17 through 18.49
Underweight	Less than 18.50
Normal range	18.50 through 24.99
Overweight	25 or greater
Preobese	25 through 29.99
Obese	30 or greater
Obese class I	30 through 34.99
Obese class II	35 through 39.99
Obese class III	40 or greater

[a] BMI is calculated as weight in kilograms divided by height in meters squared.

BOX 2.8 Proposed Mechanisms for the Association of Obesity With Chronic Kidney Disease

Physical compression of the kidneys
Renal angiotensin system activation
Hyperinsulinemia
Sympathetic activation
Overnutrition
Glomerular hyperfiltration
Proteinuria-associated kidney damage
Blood pressure elevation

Reproduced with permission from National Kidney Foundation. KDOQI clinical practice guidelines and clinical practice recommendations for diabetes and chronic kidney disease. *Am J Kidney Dis*. 2007;49(2 suppl 2):S1-S180.

Biochemical Data, Medical Tests, and Procedures

To accurately assess the ramifications of the various biochemical data that are affected by CKD, the RDN must understand the stages of CKD (see Table 1.1 on page 3) and their effect on nutrition assessment. These biochemical data are directly related to the metabolic abnormalities of CKD, including anemia, bone and mineral abnormalities, electrolyte imbalances, hyperglycemia, inflammation, protein-energy malnutrition, acid–base balance, and fluid balance. Box 2.9 relates biochemical parameters to the metabolic conditions of CKD.[17] Accepted values for each of these parameters as well as the frequency of measurements for some may change with the stage of CKD, as described in Box 2.10 on page 37 and Table 2.1 on page 43.[7,18]

BOX 2.9 Biochemical Data Used in Nutrition Assessment of Patients With Chronic Kidney Disease[17]

Anemia assessment
- Hemoglobin
- Serum transferrin saturation or reticulocyte hemoglobin content
- Mean corpuscular hemoglobin
- Mean corpuscular volume[a]
- Differential and platelet count[a]
- Serum iron
- Serum ferritin
- Total iron-binding capacity (TIBC)
- Absolute reticulocyte count
- Red blood cell folate
- Serum vitamin B12
- White blood cell count[a]

Bone health assessment
- Serum phosphorus
- Serum calcium, corrected
- Intact plasma parathyroid hormone
- Serum 25-hydroxyvitamin D

Dyslipidemia assessment
- Total cholesterol
- Low-density lipoprotein
- High-density lipoprotein
- Triglycerides

Electrolyte assessment
- Serum albumin
- Serum sodium
- Serum potassium
- Serum magnesium
- Serum carbon dioxide
- Home capillary blood glucose (CBG) records[a]

Glycemia assessment
- Home CBG records
- Hemoglobin A1c
- Serum glucose (random, fasting, preprandial, and postprandial)
- Triglycerides[a]

Continued on next page

BOX 2.9 Biochemical Data Used in Nutrition Assessment of Patients With Chronic Kidney Disease (cont.) [17]

Inflammation assessment	Serum albumin C-reactive protein White blood cell count Serum ferritin Serum iron[a] TIBC[a] Absolute reticulocyte count[a]
Kidney function assessment	Estimated glomerular filtration rate Creatinine clearance rate, 24 hours Proteinuria Proteinuria, in grams per 24 hours Urinary microalbumin-to-creatinine ratio (MAC) Glomerular filtration Serum creatinine Blood urea nitrogen Serum phosphorus Serum magnesium Cystatin C Home CBG records[a]
Protein-energy malnutrition assessment	Proteinuria Proteinuria, in grams per 24 hours Urinary MAC Serum creatinine Normalized protein nitrogen appearance Serum albumin Serum prealbumin (serum transthyretin) Home CBG records[a] Total cholesterol[a] TIBC[a]

[a] Secondary marker; additional interpretations may be appropriate.

BOX 2.10 Interpretation of Biochemical Data in Chronic Kidney Disease

Albumin

Reference range:	3.5 to 5 g/dL
Chronic kidney disease (CKD) range:	Within normal limits (WNL) for the laboratory
Interpretation of abnormal values:	High: may indicate severe dehydration
	Low: may indicate fluid overload, infection, chronic liver disease, steatorrhea, nephrotic syndrome, protein-energy malnutrition, or inflammatory gastrointestinal disease

Alkaline phosphatase

Reference range:	30 to 85 U/L
CKD range:	WNL
Interpretation of abnormal values:	High: may indicate renal osteodystrophy, malignancy, healing fractures, or liver disease
	Low: may indicate congenital hypophosphatemia or nephrotic syndrome

Aluminum

Reference range:	Less than 7 mcg/L
CKD range:	Less than 50 mcg/L
Interpretation of abnormal values:	High: may indicate ingestion of aluminum-containing medications; other possible sources of aluminum include parenteral fluids, injections, antiperspirants, or dialysates
	If more than 60 mcg/L, perform a deferoxamine test

Continued on next page

BOX 2.10 Interpretation of Biochemical Data in Chronic Kidney Disease (cont.)

Blood urea nitrogen

Reference range:	10 to 20 mg/dL
CKD range:	60 to 80 mg/dL
Interpretation of abnormal values:	High: may indicate gastrointestinal bleeding, dehydration, hypercatabolism, congestive heart failure, transplant rejection, inadequate dialysis, or excessive protein intake
	Low: may indicate liver failure, overhydration, malabsorption, acute protein intake, elevated secretion of anabolic hormones, or residual renal function

Creatinine

Reference range:	0.5 to 1.1 mg/dL for females
	0.6 to 1.2 mg/dL for males
CKD range:	2 to 15 mg/dL (based on muscle mass, glomerular filtration rate [GFR], and/or dialysis clearance)
Interpretation of abnormal values:	High: may indicate muscle damage, catabolism, myocardial infarction, acute kidney injury, CKD, inadequate dialysis, or transplant rejection
	Low: less than 10 mg/dL in chronic dialysis may indicate protein-energy malnutrition/muscle wasting or residual renal function

Ferritin

Reference range:	25 to 200 ng/mL for females
	24 to 336 ng/mL for males
CKD range:	Hemodialysis: 200 ng/mL or more
	Peritoneal dialysis: greater than 100 ng/mL

BOX 2.10 Interpretation of Biochemical Data in Chronic Kidney Disease (cont.)

Ferritin (continued)

Interpretation of abnormal values:	High: may indicate iron overload, transfusions, dehydration, or inflammatory state; values may be falsely elevated in active liver disease
	Low: may indicate iron deficiency

Folic acid

Reference range:	5 to 20 mcg/mL
CKD range:	WNL
Interpretation of abnormal values:	High: may indicate pernicious anemia or recent blood transfusions
	Low: may indicate folic acid deficiency, hemolytic anemia, malnutrition, malabsorption, malignancy, liver disease, pregnancy, alcohol use disorder, or anorexia nervosa

Glucose (fasting)

Reference range:	70 to 105 mg/dL
CKD range:	WNL
Interpretation of abnormal values:	High: may indicate diabetes, chronic hepatic disease, hyperthyroidism, malignancy, acute stress, burns, or pancreatic insufficiency
	Low: may indicate hyperinsulinemia, alcohol abuse, pancreatic tumors, liver failure, pituitary dysfunction, malnutrition, or extreme exercise

Continued on next page

BOX 2.10 Interpretation of Biochemical Data in Chronic Kidney Disease (cont.)

Hematocrit

Reference range:	37% to 47% for females
	42% to 52% for males
CKD range:	33% to 36%
Interpretation of abnormal values:	High: may indicate polycythemia or dehydration
	Low: may indicate anemias, blood loss, CKD, or insufficient erythropoiesis-stimulating agent

Intact parathyroid hormone

Reference range:	10 to 65 pg/mL
CKD range (for GFR < 15 or on dialysis):	Kidney Disease Outcomes Quality Initiative: 150 to 300 pg/mL
	Kidney Disease Improving Global Outcomes: 2 to 9 times normal limit
Interpretation of abnormal values:	High: may indicate hyperparathyroidism, nonparathyroid hormone–producing tumors, lung or kidney cancer, hypocalcemia, malabsorption, vitamin D deficiency, or rickets
	Low: may indicate hypoparathyroidism, hypercalcemia, metastatic bone tumor, sarcoidosis, vitamin D intoxication, or hypomagnesemia

Iron

Reference range:	50 to 170 mcg/dL for females
	60 to 175 mcg/dL for males
CKD range:	WNL
Interpretation of abnormal values:	High: may indicate iron overload or hemolysis
	Low: may indicate iron deficiency, decreased iron intake, or blood loss

BOX 2.10 Interpretation of Biochemical Data in Chronic Kidney Disease (cont.)

Lipoproteins

Reference range:	High-density lipoprotein (HDL): greater than 55 mg/dL for females and 45 mg/dL for males
	Low-density lipoprotein (LDL): Less than 100 mg/dL
	Very low-density lipoprotein (VLDL): 25 to 50 mg/dL
CKD range:	WNL
Interpretation of abnormal values:	High HDL: may indicate familial lipoproteinemia or excessive exercise
	High LDL/VLDL: may indicate familial lipoproteinemia, nephrotic syndrome, hypothyroidism, chronic liver disease, or poor glycemic control
	Low HDL: may indicate familial hypolipoproteinemia, hepatocellular disease, or hypoproteinemia
	Low LDL/VLDL: may indicate familial hypolipoproteinemia or hypoproteinemia due to severe burns, malabsorption, or malnutrition

Magnesium

Reference range:	1.2 to 2 mEq/L
CKD range:	WNL
Interpretation of abnormal values:	High: may indicate excessive magnesium intake from water, dialysate, magnesium-containing medications, or parenteral infusion; may also indicate dehydration
	Low: may indicate ketoacidosis, hypercalcemia, some diuretics, alcohol abuse, refeeding syndrome, diarrhea/malabsorption, or malnutrition

Continued on next page

BOX 2.10 Interpretation of Biochemical Data in Chronic Kidney Disease (cont.)

Mean corpuscular volume

Reference range: 80 to 95 µm^3

CKD range: WNL

Interpretation of abnormal values: High: may indicate folic acid or vitamin B12 deficiency, cirrhosis, reticulocytosis, chronic alcohol use disorder, or adverse effects of medications (eg, some chemotherapy agents and some immunosuppressants)

Low: may indicate chronic iron deficiency or anemia of chronic disease

Prealbumin

Reference range: 15 to 36 mg/dL

CKD range: 30 mg/dL or greater

Interpretation of abnormal values: High: may indicate use of corticosteroids

Low: may indicate liver disease, malnutrition, or inflammation

Vitamin B12

Reference range: 160 to 950 pg/mL

CKD range: WNL

Interpretation of abnormal values: High: may indicate leukemia, polycythemia vera, or severe liver dysfunction

Low: may indicate pernicious anemia, atrophic gastritis, malabsorption syndrome, inflammatory bowel disease, or vitamin C or folic acid deficiency

Adapted with permission from McCann L. *Pocket Guide to Nutrition Assessment of the Patient With Kidney Disease*. 6th ed. National Kidney Foundation; 2021.

TABLE 2.1 Frequency of Measures to Evaluate Metabolic Bone Disease in Patients With Chronic Kidney Disease[7,18]

Measure	Frequency By Chronic Kidney Disease Stage, mo		
	Progressive 3a to 3b	4	5 to 5D
Calcium and phosphorus	6-12	3-6	1-3
PTH	Baseline	6-12	3-6
Alkaline phosphatase	Baseline	6-12	12, or more frequently if PTH is elevated
Calcidiol (25-hydroxyvitamin D)	Baseline	Baseline	Baseline

Abbreviations: mo = months; PTH = parathyroid hormone

Nutrition Focused Physical Findings

The *Abridged Nutrition Care Process Terminology (NCPT) Reference Manual*[1] and the eNCPT[2] outline numerous factors to consider when gathering and interpreting nutrition focused physical findings as part of a complete nutrition assessment. Examples of potential findings in patients with CKD include the following[1,2]:

- Overall appearance: cushingoid appearance; obesity, short stature; cachexia for age
- Adipose: atrophy of orbital fat; central adiposity
- Bones: acromion abnormal prominence; clavicle abnormal prominence
- Cardiovascular-pulmonary system: edema; shortness of breath; interdialytic weight gain
- Digestive system: excessive belching; cheilosis; xerostomia; gingivitis; heartburn; ketone smell on breath; oral lesions; dry or cracked lips; altered mastication; polydipsia; stomatitis; compromised or painful swallow function; taste alteration; teeth, specify

(edentulous, partially or completely); tongue, specify (bright red, magenta, dry cracked, glossitis, impaired movement, frenulum abnormality); appetite, specify; ascites; bowel function, including flatus, specify (type, frequency, volume); epigastric pain; nausea; satiety, specify; vomiting

- Edema: anasarca; ankle edema; pitting edema
- Extremities: amputations; hypotonia; tetany
- Eyes: Bitot spots; night blindness; jaundiced sclera; xerophthalmia
- Hair: brittle; lifeless; coiled; loss; easily pluckable
- Head: altered olfactory sense, specify; temporal wasting
- Hand and nails: clubbing; Beau lines; spoon-shaped nails
- Mouth: ageusia; angular stomatitis; blue lips; dry lips; dysgeusia; gingival hypertrophy; gingivitis; halitosis; oral lesion; stomatitis; uremic breath; pale gums
- Muscles—nerves and cognition: gait disturbance; confusion
- Skin: calcinosis; dry; follicular hyperkeratosis; poor turgor; petechiae; pressure ulcers; poor wound healing; xanthomas
- Vital signs: blood pressure; heart rate; temperature

Patient History

Data to be gathered and considered in the nutrition assessment include:
- social history;
- personal medical and health history, including comorbid conditions;
- demographic information;
- treatment/therapy history; and
- family medical history, with a focus on conditions that might lead to a higher risk of kidney disease, including diabetes, hypertension, hyperlipidemia, and kidney stones.

Assessment of the patient's current level of physical activity and any known reasons that physical activity is contraindicated will also assist in developing the nutrition prescription.

Comparative Standards

In using comparative standards, "nutrition and dietetics practitioners determine, in advance, the appropriate reassessment data or nutrition care indicators that will be reviewed and identify recognized, science-based reference standards, recommendations, client goals, or baseline or previous data that will be used for comparing the data."[2] This section presents established guidelines for the following: recommended body weight, BMI, ideal/reference body weight, goal weight, percentage of ideal body weight, and adjusted body weight for patients with CKD who are obese and underweight (see Box 2.11); amputation adjustments (see Table 2.2 on page 46)[3,19]; and energy needs during acute illness (see Table 2.3 on page 47).[20]

BOX 2.11 Calculating Ideal, Standard, and Adjusted Body Weight in Patients With Chronic Kidney Disease

Ideal body weight (Hamwi method)

Females: 100 lb (45.45 kg) for first 5'0" (152 cm) and add 5 lb (2.27 kg) for each additional inch (2.54 cm) above 5'0"

Males: 106 lb (48.18 kg) for first 5'0" (152 cm) and add 6 lb (2.72 kg) for each additional inch (2.54 cm) above 5'0"

Note: Can subtract 10% for a small frame and add 10% for a large frame.

Adjusted body weight

Adjusted body weight is based on the assumption that 25% of excess body weight (adipose tissue) in patients who are obese is metabolically active tissue.

Caution: This has not been validated for use in chronic kidney disease (CKD) and may overestimate or underestimate energy and protein requirements.

If used, it is recommended that practitioners adjust body weight for calculation of nutrient recommendation if the patient's weight is less than 95% or greater than 115% of the ideal/standard body weight.

Continued on next page

BOX 2.11 Calculating Ideal, Standard, and Adjusted Body Weight in Patients With Chronic Kidney Disease (cont.)

Adjusted body weight (continued)
Adjusted body weight methods

Adjusted body weight = Ideal body weight + [(Actual body weight − Ideal body weight) × 0.25]

Adjusted body weight = Edema-free body weight + [(Standard body weight − Edema-free body weight) × 0.25]

Standard body weight
Average 50th percentile weights for males and females by age, height, and frame size in the United States are based on data from the Second National Health and Nutrition Examination Survey (NHANES). Tables are published in the 2000 Kidney Disease Outcomes Quality Initiative nutrition guideline.[a]

Caution: Although data are validated and standardized and use a large database of ethnically diverse groups, data are provided only on what individuals weigh, not what they should weigh to reduce morbidity and mortality.

Edema-free body weight
Edema-free body weight is analogous to estimated dry weight in the patient being treated by renal replacement therapies.

[a] Kidney Disease Outcomes Quality Initiative, National Kidney Foundation. Clinical practice guidelines for nutrition in chronic renal failure. *Am J Kidney Dis.* 2000;35(6 suppl 2):S17-S104. Adapted with permission from Ikizler TA, Burrowes JD, Byham-Gray LD, et al; KDOQI Nutrition in CKD Guideline Work Group. KDOQI clinical practice guideline for nutrition in CKD: 2020 update. *Am J Kidney Dis.* 2020;76(3 suppl 1):S1-S107.

TABLE 2.2 Amputation Adjustments[3,19]

Body segment	Average percentage of total body weight[a]
Entire arm	5.0
Forearm and hand	2.3
Hand	0.7
Entire leg	16.0
Lower leg, below knee	5.9
Foot	1.5

[a] Preamputation weight can be estimated by increasing the postamputation weight by the percentage listed based on the area of amputation. Preamputation weight can be used to compare weight to various standards.

TABLE 2.3 Suggested Adjustment Factors for Estimating Energy Needs[20]

Stress	Adjustment factor[a]
Acute kidney injury	1.25
Burns (based on the percentage of body surface that is burned)	
0%-20%	1-1.5
21%-40%	1.5-1.95
41%-100%	1.85-2.05
Patient is ambulatory	1.3
Chronic kidney disease stage 5	
Not on dialysis	1
Maintenance	1-1.05
Bed rest	1.1
Infection	
Mild	1
Moderate	1.2-1.4
Severe	1.4-1.6
Maintenance hemodialysis/major trauma	1.7
Malnutrition (ongoing, severe)	0.7
Soft tissue trauma	1.15
Peritonitis, soft tissue trauma	1.15
Surgery	
Elective	1
Minor/major	1.1-1.3/1.5

[a] To be multiplied by basal energy expenditure.

Case Study

Nutrition Care Process

Step 1: Assessment

> The following case study will build on the steps of the Nutrition Care Process throughout the remaining chapters of this guide. Chapter 2 presents the details necessary for nutrition assessment, Chapter 3 will list the nutrition diagnosis statements, Chapters 4 and 5 will outline the nutrition intervention, and Chapter 6 will conclude with monitoring recommendations. The details of the case study carry over from one chapter to the next, with the information pertinent to each specific chapter highlighted for clarity.

A 56-year-old female individual with CKD stage 5D on peritoneal dialysis is admitted to the hospital.

Nutrition Assessment

Food/Nutrition-Related History

Food intake
Patient consumes traditional Cambodian foods and follows traditional Cambodian meal patterns, including rice, stir-fried vegetables, and small amounts of fish, poultry, and beef. Uses fish sauce frequently. Has been consuming increased amounts of cola soft drinks to ease nausea.

Medications
HMG-CoA reductase inhibitor (statin), renal multivitamin, calcium carbonate and sevelamer with meals, calcitriol, ferrous sulfate, insulin aspart with meals, isoniazid, vitamin B6, and lansoprazole. Has missed a few days of taking medications because of current condition.

Food and nutrition knowledge/skill
Family is aware of low phosphorus and low potassium foods; is very involved.

Physical activity
Sedentary

Anthropometric Measurements

Body Composition, Growth, and Weight History

Height
150 cm (59 in)

Admit weight
74.5 kg (164 lb)

Estimated dry weight (EDW)
72 kg (has been stable)

BMI (using EDW)
32

Frame size
Medium

Ideal body weight (IBW)
62 kg; 116% IBW

Biochemical Data, Medical Tests, and Procedures

Electrolyte and renal profile
See laboratory data table.

Nutritional anemia profile
See laboratory data table.

Urine output
500 mL/24 h

Laboratory Data for Nutrition Assessment of Patient[3]

Laboratory test	Reference range	Patient result
Potassium, mmol/L	Normal: 3.4-5 Peritoneal dialysis (PD)[a]: 3.5-5.5	5.4
Blood urea nitrogen, mg/dL	Normal: 6-20 PD: >60	58
Creatinine, mg/dL	Normal: 0.7-1.3 PD: not defined	11
Glucose, mg/dL	Normal (fasting): 60-99	92
Calcium, mg/dL	Normal: 8.6-10.2	8.8
Phosphorus, mg/dL	Normal: 2.4-4.7 PD: 3.5-5.5	5.7
Albumin, g/dL	Normal: 3.5-4.7 PD: >3.5	1.6
Hemoglobin, g/dL	Normal: 13.5-17.5 PD: 10-12	9
Capillary blood glucose, mg/dL	Normal: <150	120-250
Sodium, mmol/L	Normal: 134-143	129

[a] Reference range for patients on peritoneal dialysis.

Nutrition Focused Physical Findings

- Overall appearance: abrasions on arms and neck from scratching
- Obese with central adiposity
- Bilateral ankle edema and edema of eyelid
- Diarrhea, nausea, and vomiting
- Pale conjunctiva
- Koilonychia (spoon-shaped nails)

Patient History

Personal data: Patient is 56-year-old female individual, does not speak English; children are fluent in English and are very involved and supportive.

Patient or family nutrition–oriented medical/health history: ESRD due to hypertension. History includes type 2 diabetes. Admitted to the hospital with peritonitis, pain, nausea, vomiting, and fever. Third episode of peritonitis in 2 months. Latent tuberculosis.

Treatment/therapy: Peritoneal dialysis with five exchanges per day, each 2 L 2.5% dextrose. Type 2 diabetes mellitus managed with insulin; capillary blood glucose usually less than 250 mg/dL.

References

1. Academy of Nutrition and Dietetics. *Abridged Nutrition Care Process Terminology (NCPT) Reference Manual: Standardized Terminology for the Nutrition Care Process*. Academy of Nutrition and Dietetics; 2018.

2. Academy of Nutrition and Dietetics. Electronic Nutrition Care Process Terminology (eNCPT). Accessed November 29, 2022. www.ncpro.org

3. McCann L. *Pocket Guide to Nutrition Assessment of the Patient With Kidney Disease*. 6th ed. National Kidney Foundation; 2021.

4. Franz ML, Boucher JL, Pererira RF. *Pocket Guide to Lipid Disorders, Hypertension, Diabetes, and Weight Management*. 2nd ed. Academy of Nutrition and Dietetics; 2017.

5. Uhlig K, Berns JS, Kestenbaum B, et al. KDOQI US commentary on the 2009 KDIGO clinical practice guideline for the diagnosis, evaluation, and treatment of CKD–mineral and bone disorder (CKD-MBD). *Am J Kidney Dis*. 2010;55(5):773-799. doi:10.1053/j.ajkd.2010.02.340

6. Kidney Disease: Improving Global Outcomes (KDIGO) CKD-MBD Update Work Group. KDIGO 2017 clinical practice guideline update for the diagnosis, evaluation, prevention, and treatment of chronic kidney disease–mineral and bone disorder (CKD-MBD). *Kidney Int Suppl*. 2017;7(1):1-59. doi:10.1016/j.kisu.2017.04.001

7. Kidney Disease Improving Global Outcomes (KDIGO) CKD-MBD Work Group. KDIGO clinical practice guideline for the diagnosis, evaluation, prevention, and treatment of chronic kidney disease–mineral and bone disorder (CKD-MBD). *Kidney Int Suppl*. 2009;(113):S1-S130. doi:10.1038/ki.2009.188

8. National Kidney Foundation. KDOQI clinical practice guideline for diabetes and CKD: 2012 update. *Am J Kidney Dis*. 2012;60(5):850-886. doi:10.1053/j.ajkd.2012.07.005

9. Kidney Disease Improving Global Outcomes. KDIGO clinical practice guideline for diabetes management in chronic kidney disease. *Kidney Int Suppl*. 2020;98(4S):S1-S115.

10. National Kidney Foundation. KDOQI clinical practice guidelines for managing dyslipidemias in chronic kidney disease. *Am J Kidney Dis*. 2003;41(suppl 3):S1-S92.

11. Kidney Disease Improving Global Outcomes. KDIGO clinical practice guidelines for lipid management in chronic kidney disease. *Kidney Int Suppl*. 2013;3(3):259-305.

12. National Kidney Foundation. KDOQI US commentary on the 2013 KDIGO clinical practice guideline for lipid management in CKD. *Am J Kidney Dis*. 2015;65(3):354-366. doi:10.1053/j.ajkd.2014.10.005

13. McPartland KJ, Pomposelli JJ. Update on immunosuppressive drugs used in solid-organ transplantation and their nutrition implications. *Nutr Clin Pract*. 2007;22(5):467-473. doi:10.1177/0115426507022005467

14. Ikizler TA, Burrowes JD, Byham-Gray LD, et al. KDOQI clinical practice guideline for nutrition in CKD: 2020 update. *J Kidney Dis*. 2020;76 (3 suppl 1):S1-S107. doi:10.1053/j.ajkd.2020.05.006
15. Academy of Nutrition and Dietetics Evidence Analysis Library. Recommendations summary CKD: anthropometric assessment options. 2010. Accessed November 2, 2022. www.andeal.org/topic.cfm?menu=5303
16. US Centers for Disease Control and Prevention. Defining adult overweight and obesity. CDC website. 2022. Accessed August 16, 2022. www.cdc.gov/obesity/adult/defining.html
17. Academy of Nutrition and Dietetics Evidence Analysis Library. 2020 chronic kidney disease (CKD) guideline and systematic review. 2020. Accessed August 11, 2022. www.andeal.org/topic.cfm?menu=5303
18. Inker LA, Astor BC, Fox CH, et al. KDOQI US commentary on the 2012 KDIGO clinical practice guideline for the evaluation and management of CKD. *Am J Kidney Dis*. 2014;63(5):713-735. doi:10.1053/j.ajkd.2014.01.416
19. Wiggins KL. *Guidelines for Nutrition Care of Renal Patients*. American Dietetic Association; 2001.
20. McCann L. *Pocket Guide to Nutrition Assessment of the Patient With Chronic Kidney Disease*. 4th ed. National Kidney Foundation; 2009.

CHAPTER 3

Nutrition Diagnosis

The *nutrition diagnosis* provides a formal label for the nutrition problem that has been identified from information gathered during the nutrition assessment. The diagnosis should follow the Nutrition Care Process Terminology (NCPT) for nutrition diagnoses.[1,2] As described in the Nutrition Care Process (NCP) and Nutrition Care Model, the diagnosis is based on data collected in the nutrition assessment and evaluated by the registered dietitian nutritionist (RDN) in the context of clinical experience and practice guidelines. Following the nutrition diagnosis, the next steps of the NCP are nutrition intervention (see Chapters 4 and 5) and nutrition monitoring and evaluation (see Chapter 6).

Medical diagnoses describe medical conditions that are treated by a licensed independent practitioner (eg, physician, physician assistant, or nurse practitioner). In contrast, *nutrition diagnoses* describe problems of a nutritional origin, which are clearly related to an individual's nutritional status and which are treated by nutrition interventions directed by RDNs.

The NCPT nutrition diagnosis terminology is organized into three categories[1]:

- **Intake:** actual problems related to intake of energy, nutrients, fluids, and bioactive substances through oral diet or nutrition support (ie, enteral or parenteral nutrition)
- **Clinical:** nutritional findings and/or problems that relate to medical or physical conditions

- **Behavioral-environmental:** nutritional findings or problems identified that relate to knowledge, attitudes/beliefs, physical environment, access to food, or food safety

PES Statements

After a nutrition diagnosis has been established, the RDN develops a nutrition diagnostic statement, also called a *PES (problem, etiology, signs and symptoms) statement*. This concise statement identifies the diagnosis (problem) and links it to an etiology as well as to signs and symptoms.[1,2]

A well-written PES statement follows this format: Problem *related to* etiology *as evidenced by* signs and symptoms. These terms are further defined as follows[1,2]:

- The *problem* or nutrition diagnosis term is taken from the NCPT standardized nutrition diagnosis terminology. It describes alterations in the nutrition status or contributing factors that alter the nutrition status. More than one problem may be diagnosed for a particular patient. Every problem that is identified must be addressed in the intervention and monitoring and evaluation steps of the NCP. The nutrition diagnosis terms are organized into three domains: intake, clinical, and behavioral-environmental.

- The *etiology* describes the underlying cause or contributing risk factor of the diagnosis. For example, an etiology such as "lack of prior nutrition education" suggests that the intervention will include education or counseling about the problem, whereas an etiology such as "overfeeding of parenteral/enteral nutrition" might indicate the need to adjust the nutrition support regimen. Thus, the etiology leads to an intervention. Nutrition diagnosis etiology category identification was recently added to the eNCPT and is discussed further later in this chapter.

- The *signs and symptoms* in a PES statement are defining characteristics or data elements from the assessment that support the diagnosis. Moving forward, the signs and symptoms are the parameters that will be followed to measure progress toward the goals that are established in the patient's nutrition care plan.

Writing a clear PES statement is often challenging. In a well-constructed PES statement, the assessment data support the nutrition diagnosis, etiology, signs and symptoms. When constructing a PES statement, consider the following points[2]:

- **Problem:** Can the renal RDN resolve or improve the patient's nutrition diagnosis? If there is a choice between stating two nutrition diagnoses from different domains, consider the intake nutrition diagnosis as the one more specific to the RDN.
- **Etiology:** Is the etiology the "root cause" addressed with the nutrition intervention? If addressing the etiology cannot resolve the problem, can the RDN's nutrition intervention lessen the signs and symptoms?
- **Signs and symptoms:** Will measuring the signs and symptoms show that the problem is resolved or improved? Are the signs and symptoms specific enough to measure changes and show resolution or improvement of the nutrition diagnosis?

The remainder of this chapter presents general suggestions for nutrition diagnoses and PES statements that may apply for patients with chronic kidney disease (CKD) or end-stage renal disease (ESRD). These are followed by suggested nutrition diagnoses for the case study introduced in Chapter 2.

Sample PES Statements in Chronic Kidney Disease

Boxes 3.1 through 3.3, which are arranged by NCPT nutrition diagnosis domain, offer common examples of nutrition diagnoses for patients with CKD, along with corresponding PES statements.[1,2]

BOX 3.1 Selected Intake Domain Nutrition Diagnoses for Chronic Kidney Disease[1,2]

Excessive energy intake

Definition	Energy intake that exceeds expenditure, established reference standards, or recommendations based on physiological needs.
Sample PES (problem, etiology, signs and symptoms) statement	Excessive energy intake related to energy from peritoneal dialysate plus diet as evidenced by total intake exceeding estimated needs of 25 to 35 kcal/kg/d.

Inadequate energy intake

Definition	Energy intake that is less than energy expenditure, established reference standards, or recommendations based on physiological needs.
Sample PES statement	Inadequate energy intake related to decreased appetite in patient with uremic symptoms as evidenced by average daily intake less than 50% of estimated needs.

Inadequate oral intake

Definition	Oral food/beverage intake that is less than established reference standards or recommendations based on physiological needs.
Sample PES statement	Inadequate oral intake related to poor appetite in patient with uremia as evidenced by food recall showing intake of about 50% estimated energy needs.

Excessive fluid intake

Definition	Higher intake of fluid compared to established reference standards or recommendations based on physiologic needs.
Sample PES statement	Excessive fluid intake related to patient not adjusting for reduced urine output as evidenced by patient drinking 2 to 3 L fluid per day despite urine output less than 1 L/d.

Continued on next page

> **BOX 3.1 Selected Intake Domain Nutrition Diagnoses for Chronic Kidney Disease (cont.)[1,2]**
>
> ### Increased nutrient needs (example: protein)
>
> Definition
> : Increased need for a specific nutrient compared to established reference standards or recommendations based on physiological needs.
>
> Sample PES statement
> : Increased protein needs related to increased demand for protein as evidenced by patient starting peritoneal dialysis.
>
> ### Excessive mineral intake (examples: potassium and phosphorus)
>
> Definition
> : Higher intake of a specified mineral(s) compared to established reference standards or recommendations based on physiologic needs.
>
> Sample PES statement
> : Excessive potassium intake related to patient enjoying seasonal produce as evidenced by elevated serum potassium and reported increased intake of fresh tomatoes.
>
> : Excessive phosphorus intake related to food- and nutrition-related knowledge deficit as evidenced by new diagnosis of chronic kidney disease and 24-hour food recall showing intake of multiple high-phosphorus foods at each meal.
>
> ### Excessive vitamin intake (example: vitamin C)
>
> Definition
> : Higher intake of one or more vitamins compared to established reference standards or recommendations based on physiological needs.
>
> Sample PES statement
> : Excessive vitamin C intake related to food- and nutrition-related knowledge deficit as evidenced by individual with chronic kidney disease stage 4 consuming 1,000 mg of vitamin C per day.

BOX 3.2 Selected Clinical Domain Nutrition Diagnoses for Chronic Kidney Disease[1,2]

Impaired nutrient utilization (examples: potassium and glucose)

Definition	Changes in ability to metabolize nutrients and bioactive substances.
Sample PES (problem, etiology, signs and symptoms) statement	Impaired potassium utilization related to reduced potassium excretion at estimated glomerular filtration rate (eGFR) 10 mL/min/1.73 m² as evidenced by elevated serum potassium in patient adhering to 2-g potassium diet. Impaired glucose utilization related to medication side effects as evidenced by capillary blood glucose levels greater than 180 mg/dL in posttransplant patient taking tacrolimus.

Altered nutrition-related laboratory values (example: phosphorus)

Definition	Changes in laboratory values due to body composition, medications, body system changes or genetics, or changes in ability to eliminate by-products of digestive and metabolic processes.
Sample PES statement	Altered nutrition-related laboratory value (serum phosphorus) related to changes in mineral elimination in end-stage renal disease as evidenced by elevated serum phosphorus in patient with chronic kidney disease stage 5 (predialysis) who previously controlled serum phosphorus with diet.

Food-medication interaction

Definition	Undesirable harmful interaction(s) between food and over-the-counter medications, prescribed medications, herbals, botanicals, and/or dietary supplements that diminishes, enhances, or alters the effect of nutrients and/or medications.
Sample PES statement	Food-medication interaction related to patient resuming St John's Wort post kidney transplant while taking tacrolimus for immunosuppression as evidenced by new onset of subtherapeutic tacrolimus levels.

Continued on next page

BOX 3.2 Selected Clinical Domain Nutrition Diagnoses for Chronic Kidney Disease (cont.)[1,2]

Malnutrition (undernutrition)

Definition
Inadequate intake of protein and/or energy, over a period of time, sufficient to negatively impact growth/development, and/or to result in loss of fat and/or muscle stores.

Sample PES statement
Malnutrition related to severely self-restricting protein intake to 30 g/d and 1,000 kcal/d as evidenced by unintentional weight loss (>7.5% in 3 months) and loss of orbital and triceps fat in patient who requires a minimum of 60 g protein per day and 1,800 kcal/d in chronic kidney disease stage 4.

Acute disease- or injury-related malnutrition

Definition
Moderate acute disease- or injury-related malnutrition.

Sample PES statement
Acute disease- or injury-related malnutrition related to recent weight loss following hospitalization for catheter-line infection as evidenced by mild depletion of fat in the temporal and buccal regions and mild atrophy of the calf muscle.

Unintended weight loss

Definition
Decrease in body weight that is not planned or desired.

Sample PES statement
Unintended weight loss related to food aversions as evidenced by patient's reported dislike for many foods in the last month while eGFR declined sharply.

Unintended weight gain

Definition
Weight gain more than that which is desired or planned.

Sample PES statement
Unintended weight gain related to decreased activity and peritoneal dialysate energy absorption as evidenced by 7 kg (10%) weight gain in 30 days since starting peritoneal dialysis.

BOX 3.3 Selected Behavioral-Environmental Domain Nutrition Diagnoses for Chronic Kidney Disease[1,2]

Food- and nutrition-related knowledge deficit

Definition — Incomplete or inaccurate knowledge about food, nutrition, or nutrition-related information and guidelines.

Sample PES (problem, etiology, signs and symptoms) statement — Food- and nutrition-related knowledge deficit related to no prior chronic kidney disease diet education as evidenced by patient with many questions about diet and self-report of no prior chronic kidney disease nutrition education.

Unsupported beliefs/attitudes about food or nutrition-related topics

Definition — Beliefs, attitudes, or practices about food, nutrition, and nutrition-related topics that are incompatible with sound nutrition principles, nutrition care, or disease/condition (excluding disordered eating patterns and eating disorders).

Note: *Use with caution to be sensitive to patient concerns.*

Sample PES statement — Unsupported beliefs and/or attitudes about food or nutrition-related topics related to patient with pica-like behavior and desire to consume nonfood items as evidenced by reported intense cravings and subsequent intake of one large bag of ice cubes per day and interdialytic weight gains of 5 to 7 kg.

Self-monitoring deficit

Definition — Lack of data recording to track personal progress.

Sample PES statement — Self-monitoring deficit related to patient not ready for diet-lifestyle change as evidenced by no progress on suggested monitoring tool after education and encouragement from multiple dialysis team members.

Continued on next page

> **BOX 3.3 Selected Behavioral-Environmental Domain Nutrition Diagnoses for Chronic Kidney Disease (cont.)[1,2]**
>
> **Limited adherence to nutrition-related recommendations**
>
> | | |
> |---|---|
> | definition | Lack of nutrition-related changes as per intervention agreed upon by patient or population. |
> | Sample PES statement | Limited adherence to nutrition-related recommendations related to lack of support for implementing changes as evidenced by patient's inconsistent use of phosphorus binders and rising serum phosphorus. |
>
> **Undesirable food choices**
>
> | | |
> |---|---|
> | Definition | Food and/or beverage choices inconsistent with dietary intake standards (eg, Dietary Reference Intakes), national food guidelines (eg, Dietary Guidelines for Americans, MyPlate), diet quality index standards (eg, Healthy Eating Index), or as defined in the nutrition prescription. |
> | Sample PES statement | Undesirable food choices related to patient now eating most meals in college cafeteria as evidenced by inability to select foods consistent with nutrition education for chronic kidney disease stage 5 (predialysis). |

Nutrition Diagnosis Etiology Category Identification

Etiology category identification is a new concept as of the 2020 edition of the eletcronic NCPT (eNCPT).[2] The etiology category can help the RDN identify the cause or contributing factor of a nutrition diagnosis (problem). RDNs can use the etiology category to clearly communicate known root cause of a nutrition diagnosis and link it to an effective nutrition intervention to resolve or mitigate the problem. The etiology categories are as follows[2]:

- **Beliefs–attitudes etiology:** cause or contributing risk factors related to the conviction of the truth of some nutrition-related

statement or phenomenon; feelings or emotions toward that truth or phenomenon and activities
- **Cultural etiology:** cause or contributing risk factors related to the patient's values, social norms, customs, religious beliefs, and/or political systems
- **Knowledge etiology:** cause or contributing risk factors impacting the level of understanding about food, nutrition and health, or nutrition-related information and guidelines
- **Physical function etiology:** cause or contributing risk factors related to physical ability to engage in specific tasks; may be cognitive in nature
- **Physiologic–metabolic etiology:** cause or contributing risk factors related to medical/health status that may have a nutritional impact (excludes psychological etiologies—see separate category)
- **Psychological etiology:** cause or contributing risk factors related to a diagnosed or suspected mental health/psychological problem (*Diagnostic and Statistical Manual of Mental Disorders*)
- **Social–personal etiology:** cause or contributing risk factors associated with the patient's personal and/or social history
- **Treatment etiology:** cause or contributing risk factors related to medical or surgical treatment or other therapies and management or care
- **Access etiology:** cause or contributing risk factors that affect intake and the availability of safe, healthful food, water, and food/nutrition-related supplies
- **Behavior etiology:** cause or contributing risk factors related to actions that influence achievement of nutrition-related goals

For access and behavior etiologies, a more specific root cause of the etiologies may not be known but may eventually reveal beliefs–attitudes, cultural, knowledge, physical function, psychological, social–personal, or treatment etiologies.

Nutrition Diagnosis Reference Sheet

RDNs may want to create their own reference sheet that lists the nutrition diagnoses they use most often and sample PES statements. Figure 3.1 presents an example of a chart that can be completed and used when needed. For each nutrition diagnosis, take care to use the exact NCPT nutrition diagnosis label and definition and write one or two sample PES statements based on frequently seen patients.

FIGURE 3.1 Common nutrition diagnoses in my practice				
Nutrition diagnosis	Definition	Etiologies	Signs and symptoms	Sample PES statements
1.				
2.				
3.				
4.				

Abbreviations: PES = problems, etiology, signs and symptoms

Case Study

Nutrition Care Process

Step 2: Diagnosis

> This chapter adds the nutrition diagnosis portion of the NCP to information captured in the assessment presented in Chapter 2. New information is set off from the previous material in white. This new section presents some possible nutrition diagnoses and related PES statements. Later chapters continue to develop the case with information appropriate to each step of the NCP.

A 56-year-old female individual with CKD stage 5D on peritoneal dialysis is admitted to the hospital.

Nutrition Assessment

Food/Nutrition-Related History

Food Intake
Patient consumes traditional Cambodian foods and follows traditional Cambodian meal patterns, including rice, stir-fried vegetables, and small amounts of fish, poultry, and beef. Uses fish sauce frequently. Has been consuming increased amounts of cola soft drinks to ease nausea.

Medications
HMG-CoA reductase inhibitor (statin), renal multivitamin, calcium carbonate and sevelamer with meals, calcitriol, ferrous sulfate, insulin aspart with meals, isoniazid, vitamin B6, and lansoprazole. Has missed a few days of taking medications because of current condition.

Food and Nutrition Knowledge/Skill
Family is aware of low phosphorus and low potassium foods; is very involved.

Physical activity
Sedentary

Anthropometric Measurements

Body Composition, Growth, and Weight History

Height
150 cm (59 in)

Admit weight
74.5 kg (164 lb)

Estimated dry weight (EDW)
72 kg (has been stable)

BMI (using EDW)
32

Frame size
Medium

Ideal body weight (IBW)
62 kg; 116% IBW

Biochemical Data, Medical Tests, and Procedures

Electrolyte and renal profile
See laboratory data table.

Nutritional anemia profile
See laboratory data table.

Urine output
500 mL/24 h

Laboratory Data for Nutrition Assessment of Patient[a]

Laboratory test	Reference range	Patient result
Potassium, mmol/L	Normal: 3.4-5 Peritoneal dialysis (PD)[a]: 3.5-5.5	5.4
Blood urea nitrogen, mg/dL	Normal: 6-20z PD: >60	58
Creatinine, mg/dL	Normal: 0.7-1.3 PD: not defined	11
Glucose, mg/dL	Normal (fasting): 60-99	92
Calcium, mg/dL	Normal: 8.6-10.2	8.8
Phosphorus, mg/dL	Normal: 2.4-4.7 PD: 3.5-5.5	5.7
Albumin, g/dL	Normal: 3.5-4.7 PD: >3.5	1.6
Hemoglobin, g/dL	Normal: 13.5-17.5 PD: 10-12	9
Capillary blood glucose, mg/dL	Normal: <150	120-250
Sodium, mmol/L	Normal: 134-143	129

[a] Reference range for patients on peritoneal dialysis.

Nutrition Focused Physical Findings

- Overall appearance: abrasions on arms and neck from scratching
- Obese with central adiposity
- Bilateral ankle edema and edema of eyelid
- Diarrhea, nausea, and vomiting
- Pale conjunctiva
- Koilonychia (spoon-shaped nails)

Patient History

Personal data: Patient is 56-year-old female individual, does not speak English; children are fluent in English and are very involved and supportive.

Patient or family nutrition-oriented medical/health history: ESRD due to hypertension. History includes type 2 diabetes. Admitted to the hospital with peritonitis, pain, nausea, vomiting, and fever. Third episode of peritonitis in 2 months. Latent tuberculosis.

Treatment/therapy: Peritoneal dialysis with five exchanges per day, each 2 L 2.5% dextrose. Type 2 diabetes mellitus managed with insulin; capillary blood glucose usually less than 250 mg/dL.

Nutrition Diagnosis

Intake Domain

Nutrition Diagnosis

Excessive mineral intake (sodium)

Sample PES Statement

Excessive sodium intake related to cultural food patterns as evidenced by diet recall revealing frequent use of fish sauce as well as presence of ankle and orbital edema.

Clinical Domain

Nutrition Diagnosis

Altered nutrition-related laboratory values (serum phosphorus and albumin)

Sample PES Statements

- Altered nutrition-related laboratory values (serum phosphorus) related to missed binder doses as evidenced by patient report and serum phosphorus value of 5.7 mg/dL.
- Altered nutrition-related laboratory values (serum albumin) related to altered nutrient utilization in inflammatory state as evidenced by serum albumin of 1.6 g/dL in a patient with acute peritonitis.

Behavioral-Environmental Domain

Nutrition Diagnosis

Limited adherence to nutrition-related recommendations

Sample PES Statement

Limited adherence to nutrition-related recommendations related to the use of high-phosphorus soft drinks to treat gastrointestinal symptoms as evidenced by patient reports of drinking cola beverages during episodes of nausea.

References

1. Academy of Nutrition and Dietetics. *Abridged Nutrition Care Process Terminology (NCPT) Reference Manual: Standardized Terminology for the Nutrition Care Process*. Academy of Nutrition and Dietetics; 2018.
2. Academy of Nutrition and Dietetics. Electronic Nutrition Care Process Terminology (eNCPT). Accessed November 29, 2022. www.ncpro.org

CHAPTER 4

Nutrition Intervention— Part 1: Planning the Nutrition Prescription

Nutrition intervention is the third step of the Nutrition Care Process (NCP). As stated in the Nutrition Care Process Terminology, the goal of nutrition intervention is "to resolve or improve the identified nutrition diagnosis(es) or nutrition problems by planning and implementing appropriate nutrition interventions" that are "tailored to the client's needs."[1] The nutrition diagnosis and its etiology—identified in the problem, etiology, signs and symptoms (PES) statement (see Chapter 3)—drive the selection of a nutrition intervention.[1]

The *nutrition prescription* is defined as "the client's tailored recommended dietary intake of energy and/or selected foods or nutrients based on current reference standards and evidence-based nutrition practice guidelines and related to the client's health condition and nutrition diagnosis."[1] The purpose of the nutrition prescription is to communicate the nutrition professional's diet and/or nutrition recommendation based on the nutrition assessment.[1]

Nutrition prescription recommendations in this chapter are based on the evidence-based practice guidelines listed in Chapter 1 (see Box 4.1).[1]

Nutrition Intervention—Part 1: Planning the Nutrition Prescription

This chapter reviews planning the nutrition prescription for patients with chronic kidney disease (CKD). Chapter 5 covers implementation of the nutrition prescription.

BOX 4.1 Considerations in Developing a Nutrition Prescription for Chronic Kidney Disease[1]

The nutrition intervention for chronic kidney disease (CKD) includes developing the nutrition prescription by evaluating the following:
- Energy needs based on nutrition assessment and diagnosis (eg, in kilocalories per kilogram per day)
- Carbohydrate distribution to balance estimated macronutrient needs and promote protein sparing
- Protein needs based on stage of CKD and treatment (eg, conservative management of renal disease vs renal replacement therapy) to promote normal nutritional status
- Fat distribution to balance estimated macronutrient needs, promote protein sparing, and heart health
- Vitamin intake (eg, over-the-counter supplements, fortified foods) regarding vitamins pertinent to CKD, including vitamin C, vitamin D, and others as appropriate
- Mineral intake (eg, over-the-counter supplements, fortified foods) regarding minerals pertinent to CKD, including calcium, iron, phosphorus, potassium, sodium, and others as appropriate
- Fluid intake based on fluid balance
- Fiber intake
- Cholesterol intake
- Level of bioactive substances
- Enteral or parenteral nutrition as appropriate
- Modification of texture and/or liquid consistency
- Renal diet exchanges for each food group to meet energy, protein, carbohydrate, fat, vitamin, and mineral needs

Planning the Nutrition Prescription: Chronic Kidney Disease Stages 1 Through 5 (Not on Dialysis)

Table 4.1 summarizes medical nutrition therapy (MNT) goals for patients with CKD stage 1 through 5 (not on dialysis).[2-9] The following sections provide additional information on specific nutrient requirements as well as the use of nutrition support for this patient population.

TABLE 4.1 Medical Nutrition Therapy Recommendations for Chronic Kidney Disease Stages 1 Through 5, Not on Dialysis, With or Without Diabetes[2-9]

Nutrient[a]	CKD stage	Recommendation
Energy	CKD 1-5	25-35 kcal/kg BW/d[2]
Protein	CKD 1-2, no diabetes	1.4 g/kg BW/d[3]
	CKD 3-5,[b] no diabetes, metabolically stable	0.55-0.6 g/kg BW/d; 0.28-0.43 g/kg BW/d plus ketoacid/amino acid analogs to provide 0.55-0.6 g/kg BW/d[2]
	CKD 3-5, with diabetes	0.6-0.8 g/kg BW/d, with goal to maintain nutrition status and optimize glycemic control[2]
Type of protein	CKD 1-5	Lack of evidence to recommend animal or plant protein to affect nutrition status, calcium or phosphorus levels, or lipid laboratory values[2]
Carbohydrate	CKD 1-4	50%-60% of total energy[3]
Fruit and vegetable intake	CKD 1-4	Increased intake may decrease BW, blood pressure, and net acid production[2]; avoid hyperkalemia

TABLE 4.1 Medical Nutrition Therapy Recommendations for Chronic Kidney Disease Stages 1 Through 5, Not on Dialysis, With or Without Diabetes (cont.)[2-9]

Nutrient[a]	CKD stage	Recommendation
Fiber	CKD 1-4	20-30 g/d[5]
Soluble fiber	CKD 1-4	5-10 g/d[5]
Cholesterol	CKD 1-4	<200 mg/d[3]
Total fat[c]	CKD 1-4	<30% of total energy[3]
Saturated fat	CKD 1-4	<10% of total energy[3]
PUFA	CKD 1-4	≤10% of total energy[5]
Long-chain omega-3 PUFA	CKD 3-5	2 g/d to lower serum triglyceride levels[2]
Monounsaturated fatty acid	CKD 1-4	≤20% of total energy[5]
Trans fat	CKD 1-5	Limit intake[6]
Electrolytes		
Sodium	CKD 1-2	<2.4 g/d,[7] <2 g/d with high blood pressure and diabetes[4,8]
	CKD 3-5	<2.3 g/d,[2] <2 g/d with high blood pressure and diabetes[4,8]
Phosphorus	CKD 1-2	Consider bioavailability of phosphorus sources (eg, type of food and/or food additives)[2]
	CKD 3-5	Adjust intake to maintain serum phosphorus in normal range; consider bioavailability of phosphorus sources (eg, type of food and/or food additives)[2]

Continued on next page

TABLE 4.1 Medical Nutrition Therapy Recommendations for Chronic Kidney Disease Stages 1 Through 5, Not on Dialysis, With or Without Diabetes (cont.)[2-9]

Nutrient[a]	CKD stage	Recommendation
Calcium	CKD 1-2	No evidence-based standard has been published
	CKD 3-4	800-1,000 mg/d (elemental calcium from diet intake, calcium supplements, calcium binders) for adults not taking vitamin D analogs,[2] < 2,000 mg/d from all sources[7]
	CKD 5	Avoid hypercalcemia,[9] < 2,000 mg/d from all sources[7]
Potassium	CKD 1-2	>4 g/d[3]; monitor serum potassium and adjust intake to maintain normal levels
	CKD 3-5	Adjust dietary potassium intake to maintain serum levels within normal limits; with high or low levels, base potassium intake on individual needs and clinical judgment.[2]

Abbreviations: BW = body weight; CKD = chronic kidney disease, PUFA = polyunsaturated fatty acid
[a] Emphasize whole-food sources such as fresh vegetables, whole grains, nuts, legumes, low-fat or nonfat dairy products, canola oil, olive oil, cold-water fish, and poultry.
[b] Under close clinical supervision.[2]
[c] Adjust so total energy from protein, fat, and carbohydrate are 100%.

Dietary Patterns: Chronic Kidney Disease 1 Through 5

The 2020 update of the Kidney Disease Outcomes Quality Initiative (KDOQI) clinical practice guideline for nutrition in CKD from the National Kidney Foundation and the Academy of Nutrition and Dietetics evaluates the benefits of following various dietary patterns for adults with CKD. The research literature led to the following conclusions and/or recommendations[2]:

- For adults with CKD stage 1 through 5 not on dialysis with or without dyslipidemia, "we suggest that prescribing a **Mediterranean Diet** may improve lipid profiles (2C)."
- For adults with CKD stage 1 through 4, "we suggest that prescribing **increased fruit and vegetable intake** may decrease body weight, blood pressure, and net acid production (NEAP) (2C)."

The registered dietitian nutritionist (RDN) should use clinical judgment to evaluate whether the Mediterranean diet or increased consumption of fruits and vegetables is appropriate for the individual patient based on their stage of CKD and serum potassium levels.[2]

Protein Prescription: Chronic Kidney Disease 1 Through 5

The 2020 KDOQI/Academy of Nutrition and Dietetics work group[2] reviewed the research to evaluate whether there is a benefit to consuming animal or "vegetable protein diets" on nutritional status, chronic kidney disease–mineral and bone disorder (CKD-MBD), or lipid levels. The work group[2] concluded that there was not enough evidence to promote consumption of either animal or plant protein in adults with CKD stage 1 through 5 for the stated areas of interest (1B).

Chronic Kidney Disease 3 Through 5, Without Diabetes

For metabolically stable adults with CKD stage 3 through 5 (not on dialysis) and without diabetes, the RDN should recommend or prescribe a protein-controlled diet providing 0.55 to 0.6 g dietary protein per kilogram of body weight per day "to reduce risk for end-stage kidney disease (ESKD)/death (1A) and improve quality of life (2C)."[2] Refer to Box 4.2 on page 76 for an overview of what constitutes *metabolically stable*.[2]

When recommending lower protein intakes, the RDN should use clinical judgment and consider the patient's level of motivation, willingness to participate in recommended follow-up, and risk for protein-energy malnutrition.

> **BOX 4.2   The Metabolically Stable Patient[2]**
>
> No current inflammatory process (eg, infections, cancer, transplant rejection)
> No antibiotics or immunosuppressive medications prescribed
> No hospital admissions within the past 2 weeks
> Well-controlled diabetes
> No recent, significant weight loss

Chronic Kidney Disease 3 Through 5, Without Diabetes, Very Low Protein Intake With Ketoacid/Amino Acid Analogs

A very low-protein diet may be considered for patients with CKD stage 3 through 5 when ketoacid/amino acid analogs are available and when the patient is metabolically stable "to reduce risk for end-stage kidney disease (ESKD)/death (1A) and improve quality of life (2C)."[2] The 2020 KDOQI/Academy of Nutrition and Dietetics guideline recommends "a very low-protein diet providing 0.28–0.43 g dietary protein/kg body weight/day with additional ketoacid/amino acid analogs to meet protein requirements (0.55/0.60 g/kg body weight/day)."[2] See Table 4.2 for an overview of commercially available oral ketoacid/amino acid analogs.[10]

Protein-energy wasting (PEW) is a concern in patients with CKD. Therefore, calculating and balancing adequate macronutrient intake is required when constructing diet recommendations.[2]

Chronic Kidney Disease 3 Through 5, With Diabetes

For patients with diabetic kidney disease (DKD; CKD stages 3 through 5), the RDN may prescribe a protein-controlled diet providing 0.6 to 0.8 g protein per kilogram of body weight per day (OPINION).[2] Carbohydrate and fat intake should be adjusted to promote protein sparing and glycemic control.[2]

TABLE 4.2 Commercially Available Oral Ketoacid/Amino Acid Analogs[10]

Brand (manufacturer)	Form	Dosage	Considerations
Ketorena (Nephcentric LLC, US)	Powder, vanilla flavored	1 scoop = 2,100 mg = 2.1 g KA/AA Start at 1 scoop 3 times per day (or 0.1 g/kg/d) Mix with 2-3 oz water or juice	Individualize 1 scoop is equivalent to 3-4 (600 mg) KA/AA tablets Low calcium No magnesium
Ketosteril (Fresenius Kabi India Pvt Ltd, part of Fresenius Health Care Group, Germany)	Tablet	4-8 KA/AA tablets 3 times per day with meals	May not be available in all countries Monitor serum calcium regularly Swallow whole Not for children or during pregnancy

Abbreviation: KA/AA = ketoacid analog/amino acid analog

Adapted with permission from McCann L. *Pocket Guide to Nutrition Assessment of the Patient with Kidney Disease*. 6th ed. National Kidney Foundation; 2021.

Energy Prescription: Chronic Kidney Disease 1 Through 5

It is important to use clinical judgment to determine the ideal edema-free body weight to use to calculate energy needs for patients with CKD.[7] See Chapter 2 for a full discussion on how to determine the appropriate weight for energy calculations.

For metabolically stable adults with CKD 1 through 5, the RDN should recommend an energy intake between 25 and 35 kcal per kilogram of body weight per day (1C),[2] based on the following factors[2,7]:

- weight status, body composition, and goals
- age and sex

- level of physical activity
- impact of metabolically stressing diagnoses

Research indicates that appropriate energy intakes within the recommended level assist in preventing malnutrition in adults with CKD.[2]

Once daily energy needs are determined, it is imperative to balance the intake of protein, carbohydrate, and fat to promote a healthful diet that does not include an excessive amount of any specific macronutrient.

Carbohydrate Prescription: Chronic Kidney Disease 1 Through 5

Diabetes is the leading cause of CKD in developed countries, and it is becoming the major cause of CKD in developing countries as the incidence of both diabetes and obesity increases.[3] Intensive treatment of hyperglycemia that avoids hypoglycemia can prevent DKD and may slow the progression of established kidney disease.[7]

For adults with diabetes and CKD stages 1 through 5, the RDN should implement MNT for diabetes care to manage hyperglycemia[7] and to achieve a target hemoglobin A1c (HbA1c) of approximately 6.5% to 8%.[4] The recommended HbA1c target range is associated with better overall survival. Care must be taken when evaluating HbA1c, as the accuracy and precision of HbA1c measurement declines as kidney function worsens.[4] When determining a HbA1c target for adults with DKD, evaluate the following[4]:

- stage of CKD
- macrovascular complications
- medical history
- life expectancy
- hypoglycemic awareness
- resources to treat hypoglycemic episodes
- likelihood of diabetes therapy to cause hypoglycemia

For patients with CKD and diabetes, consider limiting intake of dietary carbohydrate to 50% to 60% of calories per day (see Table 4.1).[3]

The dietary carbohydrate and fat recommendations must provide adequate energy to spare dietary protein for anabolism and to achieve and maintain a healthy weight.

Fat Prescription: Chronic Kidney Disease 1 Through 5

When determining the fat prescription, the patient's cardiovascular risk should be considered.[5] The fat prescription should set healthful targets for the amounts and types of fat to be consumed (ie, saturated, polyunsaturated, and monounsaturated) or eliminated (ie, *trans*). Daily total dietary fat and saturated fat intake should be limited to less than 30% and less than 10% of calories, respectively (see Table 4.1).[3] Decreased levels of long-chain omega-3 polyunsaturated fatty acids (PUFAs) have been found in patients with CKD, leading the 2020 KDOQI/Academy of Nutrition and Dietetics work group[2] to recommend an intake of 2 g/d to reduce elevated serum triglyceride levels.

According to the Academy of Nutrition and Dietetics evidence-based nutrition practice guidelines for CKD, "there is insufficient evidence to support fish oil therapy to improve renal function ... or graft survival for kidney transplant patients."[7] However, evidence suggests that fish oil supplementation may be beneficial in reducing oxidative stress and improving lipid profiles in adults with CKD.[7]

Micronutrient Prescription: Chronic Kidney Disease 1 Through 5

The 2020 KDOQI work group[2] reviewed the research regarding micronutrient needs of patients with CKD stage 1 through 5 and provided the following expert opinions and recommendations on vitamin and mineral intake:

- For adults with CKD stage 3 through 5, "it is reasonable for the registered dietitian nutritionist (RDN) or international equivalent to encourage eating a diet that meets the Recommended Dietary

Allowance (RDA) for adequate intake for all vitamins and minerals (OPINION)."
- For adults with CKD stage 3 through 5, "it is reasonable for the registered dietitian nutritionist (RDN) or international equivalent, in close collaboration with a physician or physician assistant, to assess dietary vitamin intake periodically and to consider multivitamin supplementation for individuals with inadequate vitamin intake (OPINION)."

Vitamin Prescription: Chronic Kidney Disease 1 Through 5

Following are vitamin recommendations for patients with CKD stage 1 through 5 (also summarized in Box 4.3 on page 82)[2,7,9,11,12]:

- **Vitamin A** supplementation is not recommended in CKD stages 3 through 5 (OPINION) because serum vitamin A and/or E levels may increase as renal function worsens.[11]
- If a patient's 25-hydroxyvitamin D serum level is less than 20 ng/mL,[10,12] **vitamin D** supplementation can be considered as follows:
  - Treat serum vitamin D insufficiency and deficiency using treatment strategies recommended for the general population.[9,13-15]
  - With vitamin D insufficiency (defined as serum vitamin D values between 12 and 20 ng/mL),[10,12] supplementation of 800 to 1,000 IU of vitamin D may be adequate.[12]
  - For vitamin D deficiency (defined as serum vitamin D <12 ng/mL),[10,12] initially treat with 50,000 IU ergocalciferol (vitamin D2) or cholecalciferol (vitamin D3) once per week, by mouth, for 6 to 8 weeks.[12] The dosage should then be reduced to 800 to 1,000 IU cholecalciferol (vitamin D3) per day.[12]
  - When treating vitamin D deficiency or insufficiency, the 2020 KDOQI guideline suggests delivering vitamin D supplementation as cholecalciferol and ergocalciferol (2C).[2]

- If an adult has nephrotic syndrome and CKD stage 1 through 5, the 2020 KDOQI guideline suggests "supplementation of cholecalciferol, ergocalciferol, or other safe and effective 25(OH)D precursors (OPINION)."[2]

- **Vitamin C** supplementation is sometimes used to improve iron absorption in adults with CKD and iron-deficiency anemia.[7] Daily vitamin C intake should be restricted to an upper limit of 90 mg/d for males and 75 mg/d for females (OPINION) (see Box 4.3 on page 82).[2] Patients with CKD are at risk of hyperoxalosis with higher doses of vitamin C.[7]

- For adults with CKD and elevated mean corpuscular volume (MCV) (eg, >100 ng/mL), the RDN should evaluate **vitamin B12** and **folic acid** levels and recommend supplementation as needed. A dietary protein restriction (≤0.6 g/kg/d) may contribute to vitamin B12 deficiency.[7] The 2020 KDOQI guideline suggests providing a folate, vitamin B12, and/or B-complex supplement to correct deficiency/insufficiency in adults with CKD stage 3 through 5 (2B) (see Box 4.3).[2] Patients with CKD have a predisposition for anemia, and all potential causes should be investigated.[7]
  - There is no evidence to support routine supplementation of folate with or without B-complex to reduce adverse cardiovascular outcomes (1A).[2]
  - Monitor patients with an estimated glomerular filtration rate (GFR) of 30 mL/min/1.73 m² or greater for vitamin B12 deficiency if they are treated with metformin for more than 4 years.[4]

- To date, no peer-reviewed research has reported the effects of micronutrients on preserving kidney function among nondialyzed adults with CKD, nephrotic syndrome, diabetic nephropathy, or kidney transplant.[7]

BOX 4.3 Recommended Micronutrients for Patients With Chronic Kidney Disease, Not on Dialysis[2,7,9,11]

Micronutrient	Daily recommendation[a]
Vitamin A	Supplementation is not recommended[11]
Vitamin D	Supplement to correct insufficiency/deficiency[2,9]
Vitamin E	15 mg[11]
Vitamin K	Males: 120 mcg[11] Females: 90 mcg[11] Avoid vitamin K supplementation in patients prescribed anticoagulant medications[2]
Vitamin C	For adults at risk of deficiency, supplement starting as follows: Males: 90 mg[2,7] Females: 75 mg[2,7]
Thiamin (vitamin B1)	Males aged 50 to 70 years: 1.2 mg[11] Females aged 50 to 70 years: 1.1 mg[11]
Riboflavin (vitamin B2)	Males: 1.3 mg[11] Females: 1.1 mg[11]
Niacin (vitamin B3)	Males: 16 mg[11] Females: 14 mg[11]
Pyridoxine (vitamin B6)	5 mg[11]
Folic acid	Chronic kidney disease (CKD) stage 1 through 5: supplement to correct insufficiency/deficiency[2] CKD stage 3 through 5: no routine supplementation with hyperhomocysteinemia[2]

BOX 4.3	Recommended Micronutrients for Patients With Chronic Kidney Disease, Not on Dialysis (cont.)[2,7,9,11]
Micronutrient	*Daily recommendation[a]*
Cobalamin (vitamin B12)	CKD stage 1 through 5: supplement to correct insufficiency/deficiency[2]
Pantothenic acid (vitamin B5)	Aged 51 years or more: 5 mg = Adequate Intake[11]
Selenium	No routine supplementation[2]
Zinc	No routine supplementation[2]

[a] Recommendations are for both males and females unless otherwise specified.

Electrolyte and Mineral Prescription: Chronic Kidney Disease 1 Through 5

Sodium

Limiting sodium intake to less than to 2.3 g/d (1B) is recommended for patients with CKD stage 3 through 5 to improve blood pressure and volume control/fluid balance.[2] For patients with CKD stage 3 through 5 with high blood pressure and diabetes, evidence-based guidelines recommend reducing sodium intake to less than 2 g/d.[4,8] A sodium-limiting diet may also impact fluid volume and body weight in adults with CKD stage 3 through 5 (2B).[2] Sodium intake should be adjusted as appropriate based on the patient's fluid balance, blood pressure control, and other clinical findings.[7] For instance, a diet restricted in sodium may not be appropriate for patients with sodium-wasting nephropathy.[8]

For adults with CKD stage 3 through 5 and proteinuria, the 2020 KDOQI work group found enough data to recommend "limiting dietary sodium intake to less than 2.3 g/d to reduce proteinuria synergistically with available pharmacologic interventions (2A)."[2]

Management of Acid Load

Maintaining acid-base balance becomes more difficult as kidney function declines. Dietary protein intake influences acid load. A higher protein intake results in a higher acid load.[2] The 2020 KDOQI guideline recommends supplementing a bicarbonate or a citric acid/sodium citrate solution to decrease NEAP and preserve renal function for adults with CKD stage 3 through 5 (1C).[2] Consider maintaining serum bicarbonate between 24 and 26 mmol/L in adults with CKD stage 3 through 5 (OPINION).[2]

For adults with CKD stage 1 through 4, experts recommend increasing intake of fruits and vegetables to decrease NEAP and preserve kidney function (2C).[2] As kidney disease progresses, specifically in CKD stage 4 or higher, it is harder for the kidneys to regulate potassium excretion. When the RDN recommends a higher intake of fruits and vegetables, close monitoring of serum potassium should occur to prevent hyperkalemia.[2]

Potassium

The 2020 KDOQI guideline suggests that for adults with CKD stage 3 through 5 (2D) with either hyperkalemia or hypokalemia, "dietary or supplemental potassium intake be based on a patient's individual needs and clinician judgment."[2] If a patient with CKD stage 3 through 5 has hyperkalemia, several clinical factors should be reviewed, including trends in serum potassium levels, medications that may affect potassium, glycemic control, and dietary issues.[2,7] When evaluating hyperkalemia initially, the RDN should look at blood glucose levels and medications that may be contributing to the elevated potassium levels. Medication adjustments should be pursued prior to restricting dietary potassium. If elevated potassium levels persist despite improved blood glucose control and medication changes, dietary intake can be reviewed to pinpoint the possible or potential high potassium food choices. The RDN can advise lower potassium fruit and vegetable substitutions that continue to provide the patient with fiber and micronutrients.[2]

In addition to the above guidance, the RDN may recommend adjusting dietary potassium intake to maintain serum potassium within normal limits for adults with CKD stage 3 through 5 (OPINION).[2] The RDN should also consider that diets which may be higher in potassium, such as the Dietary Approaches to Stop Hypertension (DASH) diet, and potassium-containing salt substitutes "may not be appropriate for patients with advanced CKD or those with hyporeninemic, hypoaldosteronism or other causes of impaired potassium excretion because of the potential for hyperkalemia."[8] Hypokalemia or hyperkalemia can have a direct effect on cardiac function, with potential for cardiac arrhythmia and sudden death.[7]

Calcium

For adults with stage 3 and 4 CKD (2B) who are not prescribed vitamin D analogs, a total elemental calcium intake (including dietary calcium, calcium supplementation, and calcium-based phosphate binders) of 800 to 1,000 mg/d is recommended to maintain serum calcium levels.[2] For patients with CKD stage 5, the goal is to avoid hypercalcemia and limit total calcium intake to 2,000 mg/d from all sources.[7] Patients with CKD have a predisposition for mineral and bone disorders. Serum calcium concentration is an important factor in regulating parathyroid hormone (PTH) secretion and therefore affects bone integrity and soft tissue calcification. The RDN should be aware of the risks of hypercalcemia, including soft tissue calcification.[7]

Phosphorus

Hyperphosphatemia begins to appear when the GFR drops below 45 mL/min/1.73 m^2.[2] Because CKD-MBD is common in patients with CKD, phosphorus control is essential for the treatment and prevention of secondary hyperparathyroidism, renal bone disease, and soft tissue calcification.[7]

For adults with CKD stage 3 through 5 (1B), dietary phosphorus intake should be evaluated, and recommendations for adjusting phosphorus intake should be made to achieve serum phosphorus within normal levels. A patient's diet history can be assessed to evaluate the bioavailability of phosphorus in the foods as well as any consumed phosphorus additives when developing the diet recommendations (OPINION).[2]

For adults with CKD stage 3 through 5, the dose and timing of phosphate binders should be adjusted to the phosphate content of meals and snacks to achieve desired serum phosphorus levels. Serum phosphorus levels are difficult to control with dietary restrictions alone. Treatment to manage serum phosphorus should be individualized and may include dietary phosphate restriction, phosphate binders, calcium and vitamin D supplementation, and self-management training.[7]

Aluminum

Aluminum-containing antacid medications (eg, aluminum hydroxide) may cause blood or blood serum levels of aluminum to rise in patients with CKD; therefore, long-term use should be avoided.[9]

Iron

When adults with CKD have serum ferritin levels less than 500 ng/mL with serum transferrin saturation (TSAT) less than 30%, oral or intravenous iron supplementation may be recommended.[16] The amount of iron supplementation recommended should maintain levels of serum iron that will adequately support erythropoiesis.[7,16] Iron absorption may be impaired by other medications, such as phosphate binders.[7]

Magnesium

There are currently no evidenced-based guidelines that evaluate the appropriate daily intake of magnesium for patients with CKD.[7] Magnesium-containing antacid medications (eg, Maalox and Phillips' Milk of Magnesia) may cause blood or blood serum levels of magnesium to rise in patients with CKD.[17]

Zinc

Zinc intake for adults with CKD should mirror the RDA for the general population.[2] Daily nutritional intake of 8 to 12 mg elemental zinc for females and 10 to 15 mg for males is recommended.[18] When a patient's zinc intake is chronically inadequate and the patient has symptoms of zinc deficiency (impaired taste or smell, skin fragility, impotence, or peripheral neuropathy), daily supplementation with 50 mg elemental zinc for 3 to 6 months may be considered.[18] At that time, biochemical levels should be rechecked, and zinc supplementation should be discontinued if serum levels have normalized.[18]

Zinc supplementation, in high doses or over a long period of time, may lead to copper deficiency, which, if undiagnosed, may cause irreversible neurologic conditions.[19] The 2020 KDOQI guideline does not recommend routine zinc supplementation (2C).[2] RDNs should be familiar with signs and symptoms of zinc deficiency in order to recommend and monitor supplementation when needed.

Selenium

Selenium intake for adults with CKD should mirror the RDA for the general population.[2] Daily intake of 55 mcg selenium is appropriate,[18] but the 2020 KDOQI guideline does not recommend routine selenium supplementation (2C).[2] It may be appropriate for patients on hemodialysis with symptoms of selenium deficiency (eg, cardiomyopathy, skeletal myopathy, thyroid dysfunction, hemolysis, or dermatosis) to take selenium supplements for 3 to 6 months.[18] RDNs should be familiar with signs and symptoms of selenium deficiency in order to recommend and monitor supplementation when needed.[2]

Nutritional Supplementation: Chronic Kidney Disease 1 Through 5

To develop strategies that combat PEW in patients with CKD, the 2020 KDOQI work group reviewed current research and determined guidance for oral nutritional supplementation (ONS), enteral nutrition, and parenteral nutrition (PN).

Oral Nutrition Supplements

Patients with CKD may struggle to meet recommended calorie and protein needs despite receiving regular diet counseling from a renal RDN.[2] The 2020 KDOQI guideline states that for adults with CKD stage 3 through 5 (2D) at risk of or with PEW, "we suggest a minimum of a 3-month trial of oral nutritional supplements to improve nutritional status if dietary counseling alone does not achieve sufficient energy and protein intake to meet nutritional requirements."[2]

Enteral Nutrition Prescription

Patients with renal failure who require nutrition support therapy should receive enteral nutrition if their intestinal function permits it.[20] Macronutrient, vitamin, and mineral guidelines for CKD may apply to the enteral prescription.[21] The patient's serum concentrations of potassium, magnesium, phosphorus, and calcium should be monitored, and electrolyte intake can be adjusted appropriately.[20]

The 2020 KDOQI guideline suggests that in adults with CKD stage 1 through 5 (OPINION) "with chronically inadequate intake and whose protein and energy requirements cannot be attained by dietary counseling and oral nutrition supplements, it is reasonable to consider a trial of enteral tube feeding."[2]

Parenteral Nutrition Prescription

If altered gastrointestinal function prevents the patient from taking enteral nutrition, PN should be considered to support nutritional status. Macronutrient, vitamin, and mineral guidelines for CKD apply to the parenteral formula prescription. Tables 4.3[22] and 4.4[22] provide examples of formulas that may be used when PN is warranted.

TABLE 4.3 Sample Parenteral Nutrition Formulations[22]

Component	Peripheral parenteral nutrition	Standard parenteral nutrition	Concentrated parenteral nutrition
Carbohydrate, g/L[a]	100 (10% dextrose)	200 (20% dextrose)	200 (20% dextrose)
Amino acids, g/L[b]	35 (3.5% amino acids)	50 (5% amino acids)	75 (7.5% amino acids)
Electrolytes	Adjust per metabolic profile	Adjust per metabolic profile	Adjust per metabolic profile

[a] Carbohydrate: 3.4 kcal/g.
[b] Amino acids: 4 kcal/g.

TABLE 4.4 Sample Intravenous Fat Emulsions for Parenteral Nutrition[22]

Lipid concentration, %	Volume, mL	Energy, kcal/mL	Total energy, kcal
10	500	1.1	550
20	250	2	500
20	500	2	1,000

The 2020 KDOQI guideline states that for adults with CKD with PEW, "we suggest a trial of PN for CKD 1–5 patients (2C) ... to improve and maintain nutritional status if nutritional requirements cannot be met with existing oral and enteral intake."[2]

When determining PN recommendations for patients who are critically ill, the goals are as follows[22]:

1. Maintain a glucose oxidation rate of 4 mg/kg/min or less.
2. Limit intravenous fat emulsion to 1 g/kg/d.

Refer to Box 4.4[23] for a suggested composition of PN for adults with CKD.

BOX 4.4 Suggested Composition of Parenteral Nutrition Solution for Adults With Chronic Kidney Disease[23]

Macronutrient

Energy Chronic kidney disease (CKD) stage 1 through 5: 25 to 35 kcal/kg/d

Amino acids[a] CKD 3 through 5 not on hemodialysis (HD): 0.6 to 0.8 g/kg/d without diabetes; 0.8 to 0.9 g/kg/d with diabetes

CKD on chronic dialysis or peritoneal dialysis: 1 to 1.2 g/kg/d

Dextrose Consider all sources of dextrose (intravenous fluids, dialytic therapy)

Continued on next page

BOX 4.4 Suggested Composition of Parenteral Nutrition Solution for Adults With Chronic Kidney Disease (cont.)[23]

Macronutrient (continued)

Lipids	Less than 1 g/kg/d, less than 0.11 g/kg/min, or 20% to 30% of total kilocalories
	Include propofol infusion (1.1 kcal/mL) in lipid sources
	Peripheral parenteral nutrition (PN) lipid content should not exceed 60% of total kilocalories
Fluid	Volume depends on patient tolerance/requirements, insensible losses, and urine output

Micronutrients

Minerals

May need to restrict for CKD not on HD or with intermittent HD; monitor serum levels and adjust accordingly.

Higher/lower needs may occur with continuous renal replacement therapy (CRRT); varies by dialysate mineral content.

Sodium	1 to 2 mEq/kg/d standard PN
	May be removed from PN for CRRT
Potassium	1 to 2 mEq/kg/d standard PN
	May be removed from PN for CRRT
Phosphorus	20 to 40 mmol/d standard PN
	May need supplementation during CRRT
Calcium	10 to 15 mEq/d standard PN
	May need supplementation during CRRT
Magnesium	8 to 20 mEq/d standard PN
	May need supplementation during CRRT
Chloride and acetate	Proportions vary depending on acid/base status and degree of renal impairment

BOX 4.4 Suggested Composition of Parenteral Nutrition Solution for Adults With Chronic Kidney Disease (cont.)[23]

Vitamins

Standard PN regimen typically contains 10 mL multivitamin.

Supplemental B-vitamin complex or renal multivitamin may be used for deficiency in CKD.

Vitamin A	990 mcg/d or 3,300 IU
Vitamin D	5 mcg/d or 200 IU
Vitamin E	10 mg/d or 10 IU
Vitamin K	150 mcg/d
Vitamin C	200 mg/d
Thiamin (B1)	6 mg/d
Riboflavin (B2)	3.6 mg/d
Niacin (B3)	40 mg/d
Pyridoxine (B6)	6 mg/d
Cyanocobalamin (B12)	5 mcg/d
Folate	600 mcg/d
Pantothenic acid	15 mg/d
Biotin	60 mcg/d

Trace elements

Standard PN regimen typically contains a multitrace element product.

Zinc	2.5 to 5 mg/d
Copper	0.3 to 0.5 mg/d
Chromium	10 to 15 mcg/d

Continued on next page

> **BOX 4.4 Suggested Composition of Parenteral Nutrition Solution for Adults With Chronic Kidney Disease (cont.)[23]**
>
> **Trace elements (continued)**
> | | |
> |---|---|
> | Manganese | 0.06 to 0.1 mg/d |
> | Selenium | 20 to 60 mcg/d |

Adapted with permission from Glick-Bauer M, Moore E. Parenteral nutrition in kidney disease. In: Phillips S, Gonyea J, eds. *A Clinical Guide to Nutrition Care in Kidney Disease*. 3rd ed. Academy of Nutrition and Dietetics; 2022:328-329.
[a] Consider if patient is metabolically stable when determining protein needs.

Planning the Nutrition Prescription: Maintenance Hemodialysis and Peritoneal Dialysis in Chronic Kidney Disease Stage 5D

Box 4.5 summarizes MNT recommendations for patients receiving maintenance hemodialysis (MHD) or peritoneal dialysis (PD).[2,4,10,18,24] The following sections provide additional information about specific nutrient requirements as well as the use of nutrition support.

Protein Prescription: Chronic Kidney Disease 5D

The 2020 KDOQI work group reviewed the research to evaluate whether there is a benefit to consuming animal or vegetable protein diets on nutritional status, CKD-MBD, or lipid levels. The work group concluded that there was not enough evidence to promote consumption of animal or plant protein, in adults receiving MHD or PD, for the stated areas of interest (1B). The RDN should review the patient's protein intake and provide guidance on consuming adequate protein and essential amino acids to meet estimated needs.[2]

BOX 4.5 Maintenance Hemodialysis and Peritoneal Dialysis Medical Nutrition Therapy Recommendations[2,4,10,18,24]

Nutrient	Recommendation
Energy	Metabolically stable maintenance hemodialysis (MHD) and peritoneal dialysis (PD): 25 to 35 kcal/kg body weight (BW)/d[2] Acute illness MHD and PD: • Aged less than 60 y, starting at 35 kcal/kg/d[24] • Aged 60 y or older, starting at 30 to 35 kcal/kg/d[24]
Protein	Metabolically stable: • MHD and PD (without diabetes): 1 to 1.2 g/kg BW/d[2] • MHD and PD (with diabetes): 1 to 1.2 g/kg BW/d; with hyperglycemia consider higher protein intake to control blood glucose[2,4] Acute illness: • MHD: Start at 1.2 g/kg/d[24] • PD: Start at 1.3 g/kg/d[24]
Carbohydrate, total fat, and saturated fat	MHD and PD: Adjust to promote glycemic and lipid control
Long-chain omega-3 polyunsaturated fatty acid (fish oil, flaxseed, or other oils)	MHD: 1.3 to 4 g/d to decrease triglycerides and low-density lipoprotein and increase high-density lipoprotein values. Routine supplementation to decrease mortality, decrease cardiovascular events, or promote arteriovenous graft/fistula patency is not recommended.[2] PD: 1.3 to 4 g/d to improve lipid levels. Routine supplementation to decrease mortality and cardiovascular events is not recommended.[2] See Box 4.6 for expanded review
Fluid	MHD: Interdialytic weight gain less than 4% BW[10] PD: Evidence-based guidelines have not been established

Continued on next page

> **BOX 4.5 Maintenance Hemodialysis and Peritoneal Dialysis Medical Nutrition Therapy Recommendations (cont.)** [2,4,10,18,24]
>
> | Nutrient | Recommendation |
> | --- | --- |
> | **Electrolytes** | |
> | Potassium (K) | MHD and PD: Adjust K intake to maintain serum K within normal limits; with high or low K, base K intake on individual needs and clinical judgment[2] |
> | Sodium | MHD and PD: less than 2.3 g/d to reduce blood pressure and improve fluid balance. Limit sodium intake to control fluid balance and achieve a healthy BW[2] |
> | Calcium (Ca) | MHD and PD: To avoid high Ca levels, adjust Ca intake based on prescribed dose of vitamin D analogs and calcimimetics[2] |
> | Phosphorus | MHD and PD: Adjust intake to maintain serum phosphorus in normal range; consider bioavailability of oral phosphorus sources (eg, food or food additive)[2] |
> | **Micronutrients** | |
> | Vitamin D | MHD and PD: Deficiency/insufficiency, supplement with cholecalciferol or ergocalciferol[2] |
> | Multivitamin supplement | MHD and PD: See Box 4.7 |

Maintenance Hemodialysis, Without Diabetes

For metabolically stable patients receiving MHD, the 2020 KDOQI work group recommends a protein intake of 1 to 1.2 g per kilogram of body weight per day (1C).[2] If a patient undergoing MHD is acutely ill, the optimum protein intake is at least 1.2 g/kg/d.[24]

Peritoneal Dialysis, Without Diabetes

For metabolically stable patients on PD, a protein intake of 1 through 1.2 g/kg body weight/d is recommended (OPINION).[2] If the protein status of a patient on PD is depleted despite a protein intake of 1 to 1.2 g/kg body weight/d, then 1.3 g protein/kg/d could be recommended.[24] If a patient on PD is acutely ill, the optimum protein intake is at least 1.3 g/kg/d.[24]

Clinical judgment should be used to evaluate whether patients with peritonitis, malnutrition, or other metabolic stress need increased amounts of dietary protein.[25]

Maintenance Hemodialysis and Peritoneal Dialysis, With Diabetes

For metabolically stable patients with DKD, a protein intake of 1 to 1.2 g per kilogram of body weight per day is recommended (OPINION).[2] If hypoglycemia or hyperglycemia is possible, practitioners should consider higher protein intake to control blood glucose levels[3] or if chronic disease-related malnutrition is present.[26]

Energy Prescription: Chronic Kidney Disease 5D

The patient on dialysis should be prescribed an edema-free body weight or estimated dry weight. This weight prescription may be based on clinical findings (eg, blood pressure, weight gain between treatments, and symptoms such as headaches or cramps), bioimpedance measurements, or continuous blood volume monitoring or it may be determined using other assessment tools.[27,28] This dry weight represents the patient's target weight after a dialysis treatment, and it may be used for calculations of energy needs in HD and PD. Please see Chapter 2 for additional information regarding the appropriate patient weight to use for nutrient calculations.

The 2020 KDOQI guideline recommends a daily energy intake for metabolically stable patients on MHD or PD of 25 to 35 kcal per kilogram of body weight per day (1C).[2] For patients with acute illness, previous evidence-based guidelines recommend 35 kcal/kg/d for patients aged younger than 60 years and 30 to 35 kcal/kg/d for patients aged 60 years or older as a minimum starting point.[24]

For patients receiving PD, it is also necessary to adjust the energy prescription to account for the dextrose-based energy absorbed from the dialysate (Table 4.5).[10,29]

TABLE 4.5 Dextrose Contribution of Peritoneal Dialysis Solutions[10,29,a]

Percent dextrose	1 L, g[b]	2 L, g	2.5 L, g	3 L, g
1.5%	15	30	45	60
2.5%	25	50	62.5	75
4.25%	42.5	85	106.25	127.5

[a] Continuous ambulatory peritoneal dialysis = 60% to 70% dextrose absorption; continuous cyclic peritoneal dialysis = 40% to 50% dextrose absorption; ambulatory peritoneal dialysis = 30% to 50% dextrose absorption. See sample calculation in the case study at the end of Chapter 4.
[b] Each gram of dextrose provides 3.4 kcal/g.

Carbohydrate Prescription: Chronic Kidney Disease 5D

In the renal diet, carbohydrate and fat should deliver adequate energy to ensure that protein is used for physiologic functions. Carbohydrate intake needs to be sufficient without being excessive.[3] Any additional protein provided by carbohydrate foods should also be included in the total daily protein calculations for the renal diet.[25]

The dextrose provided by the peritoneal dialysate solution must be considered when managing blood glucose control for patients with diabetes who are receiving PD. To prevent unwanted weight gain and to optimize diabetic control, PD exchanges should be done with the lowest dextrose solutions that provide effective dialysis adequacy. The calories provided by the PD exchanges should be subtracted from the patient's estimated total daily energy requirements to avoid providing excess calories.

Care must be taken when evaluating HbA1c for patients with diabetes, as the accuracy and precision of HbA1c measurement declines as kidney function worsens.[4]

Fat Prescription: Chronic Kidney Disease 5D

When developing a nutrition prescription, the cardiovascular disease risk profile of patients with CKD must be considered.[30] The fat prescription should set healthful targets for the amounts and types of fat to be consumed (ie, saturated, polyunsaturated, and monounsaturated) or eliminated (ie, *trans*), with the goal of improving the patient's lipid profile.

The 2020 KDOQI work group assessed the benefits of long-chain omega-3 PUFAs for the dialysis population, which are summarized in Box 4.6.[2]

BOX 4.6 Long-Chain Omega-3 Polyunsaturated Fatty Acids in the Adult Dialysis Population[2]

Chronic kidney disease stage 5D on maintenance hemodialysis	Evidence grade	Chronic kidney disease stage 5D on peritoneal dialysis	Evidence grade
"We suggest not routinely prescribing long-chain omega-3 polyunsaturated fatty acid (LC n-3 PUFA) … to lower risk of **mortality**…"	2C	"It is reasonable not to routinely prescribe LC n-3 PUFA[a]… to lower risk of **mortality**…"	OPINION
"We suggest not routinely prescribing LC n-3 PUFA to lower risk of … **cardiovascular events**."	2B	"It is reasonable not to routinely prescribe LC n-3 PUFA … to lower risk of … **cardiovascular events**."	OPINION

Continued on next page

BOX 4.6 Long-Chain Omega-3 Polyunsaturated Fatty Acids in the Adult Dialysis Population (cont.)[a]

Chronic kidney disease stage 5D on maintenance hemodialysis	Evidence grade	Chronic kidney disease stage 5D on peritoneal dialysis	Evidence grade
"We suggest that 1.3 to 4 g/d LC n-3 PUFA may be prescribed to **reduce triglyceride and low-density lipoprotein cholesterol**…"	2C	"It is reasonable to consider prescribing 1.3 to 4 g/d LC n-3 PUFA to improve lipid profile."	OPINION
"We suggest that 1.3 to 4 g/d LC n-3 PUFA may be prescribed to … **raise high-density lipoprotein levels**."	2D	Data not available.	Data not available.
"We suggest not routinely prescribing fish oil to improve primary patency rates in patients with **arteriovenous grafts**…"	2B	Data not available.	Data not available.
"We suggest not routinely prescribing fish oil to improve primary patency rates in patients with … **fistulas**."	2A	Data not available.	Data not available.

[a] Including those derived from fish or flaxseed and other oils.[2]

Micronutrient Prescription: Chronic Kidney Disease 5D

The 2020 KDOQI work group[2] reviewed the research regarding micronutrient needs of the patient with kidney disease and provided the following expert opinions and recommendations for vitamin and mineral intake:

- For adults with CKD stage 5D, "it is reasonable for the registered dietitian nutritionist (RDN) or international equivalent to encourage eating a diet that meets the recommended dietary allowance (RDA) for adequate intake for all vitamins and minerals (OPINION)."
- For adults with CKD stage 5D, "it is reasonable for the registered dietitian nutritionist (RDN) or international equivalent, in close collaboration with a physician or physician assistant, to assess dietary vitamin intake periodically and to consider multivitamin supplementation for individuals with inadequate vitamin intake (OPINION)."
- For adults with CKD stage 5D "who exhibit inadequate dietary intake for sustained periods of time, it is reasonable to consider supplementation with multivitamins, including all the water-soluble vitamins, and essential trace elements to prevent or treat micronutrient deficiencies (OPINION)."

Vitamin Prescription: Chronic Kidney Disease 5D

Patients on dialysis should take a renal multivitamin daily to replace water-soluble vitamins that are lost in the dialysis process.[2,18] Vitamin recommendations for different situations are included in Box 4.7 on page 100.[2,18] Professional judgment should be used regarding supplementation in cases of malabsorption or vitamin deficiency and to prevent toxicity, as follows:

BOX 4.7 Daily Vitamin Recommendations for Hemodialysis[2,18]

Vitamin	Recommendation
Vitamin A	Due to potential for toxicity, do not routinely supplement[2]
Vitamin D	Supplement following strategies for the general population[2]
Vitamin E	Due to potential for toxicity, do not routinely supplement[2]
Vitamin K	Avoid vitamin K supplements in patients prescribed anticoagulant medicines[2]
Vitamin C	For adults at risk for deficiency, supplement starting at the following[2]: • Females: 75 mg • Males: 90 mg
Thiamin (vitamin B1)	Supplement: 1.1 to 1.2 mg[18] to correct for deficiency/insufficiency[2]
Riboflavin (vitamin B2)	Supplement: 1.1 to 1.3 mg[18] to correct for deficiency/insufficiency[2]
Niacin (vitamin B3)	Supplement: 14 to 16 mg[18] to correct for deficiency/insufficiency[2]
Pyridoxine (vitamin B6)	Supplement: 10 mg[18] to correct for deficiency/insufficiency[2]
Folic acid	Supplement: 1 mg[18] to correct for deficiency/insufficiency[2]
Cobalamin (vitamin B12)	Supplement: 2.4 mcg[18] to correct for deficiency/insufficiency[2]
Pantothenic acid (vitamin B5)	Supplement: 5 mg[18] to correct for deficiency/insufficiency[2]
Biotin	Supplement: 30 mcg[18]

- **Vitamin A** and **vitamin E** supplementation is not recommended for patients with CKD stage 5D (OPINION) because serum vitamin A and/or E levels may increase as renal function worsens and lead to toxicity. If vitamin A or E supplementation is needed, avoid excessive doses; patients should be monitored for toxicity (OPINION).[2]
- If a patient's serum level of 25-hydroxyvitamin D is less than 20 ng/mL,[10,12] **vitamin D** supplementation may be recommended as follows:
  - Treat serum vitamin D insufficiency and deficiency using treatment strategies recommended for the general population.[9,13-15]
  - For vitamin D insufficiency, defined as serum vitamin D values between 12 and 20 ng/mL,[10,12] supplementation of 800 to 1,000 IU of vitamin D may be adequate.[12]
  - For vitamin D deficiency, defined as serum vitamin D less than 12 ng/mL,[10,12] initially treat with 50,000 IU ergocalciferol (vitamin D2) or cholecalciferol (vitamin D3) once a week, by mouth, for 6 to 8 weeks. The dosage should then be reduced to 800 to 1,000 IU cholecalciferol (vitamin D3) per day.[12]
  - When treating vitamin D deficiency or insufficiency, the 2020 KDOQI guideline suggests delivering vitamin D supplementation as cholecalciferol and ergocalciferol (2C).[2]
- **Vitamin C** supplementation is sometimes used to improve iron absorption in adults with CKD and iron-deficiency anemia.[7] Daily vitamin C intake should be restricted to an upper limit of 90 mg/d for males and 75 mg/d for females (OPINION).[2] Patients with CKD are at risk of hyperoxalosis at higher vitamin C doses.[7]
- For adults with CKD and elevated MCV, the RDN should evaluate **vitamin B12** and **folic acid** levels and recommend supplementation as needed. The 2020 KDOQI guideline suggests providing a folate, vitamin B12, and/or B-complex supplement to correct deficiency/insufficiency in adults with CKD stage 5D (2B).[2] Patients with CKD have a predisposition for anemia, and all potential causes should be investigated.[7]
- There is no evidence to support routine supplementation of folate with or without B-complex to reduce adverse cardiovascular outcomes (1A).[2]

Electrolyte and Mineral Prescription: Chronic Kidney Disease 5D

Sodium

Limiting sodium intake to 2.3 g/d (1C) is recommended for patients with CKD stage 5D to improve blood pressure and volume control/fluid balance.[2] For patients with CKD stage 5D, high blood pressure, and diabetes, consider limiting sodium intake to 2 g/d.[4,8] A sodium-limiting diet may also impact fluid volume and body weight in adults with CKD stage 5D (2B).[2] Sodium intake should be adjusted as appropriate based on the patient's fluid balance, blood pressure control, and other clinical findings.[7]

Management of Acid Load

Maintaining acid-base balance becomes more difficult as kidney function declines.[2] Dietary protein intake influences acid load. A higher protein intake results in a higher acid load.[2] The 2020 KDOQI guideline recommends supplementing a bicarbonate or a citric acid/sodium citrate solution to reduce the rate of decline of residual kidney function and NEAP for adults with CKD stage 5D (1C).[2] Consider maintaining serum bicarbonate between 24 and 26 mmol/L in adults with CKD stage 5D (OPINION).[2]

Potassium

When a patient with CKD stage 5D presents with hyperkalemia, several clinical factors should be reviewed, including serum potassium levels, medications that may affect potassium, glycemic control, and dietary issues.[2,7] When evaluating hyperkalemia initially, the RDN should evaluate blood glucose levels and medications that may be contributing to elevated potassium levels.[2] Medication adjustments should be pursued prior to restricting dietary potassium.[2] If elevated potassium persists despite improved blood glucose control and medication changes, dietary intake should be assessed to pinpoint the possible or potential high potassium food choices. The RDN can advise lower potassium fruit and vegetable substitutions that continue to provide the patient with fiber and micronutrients.[2]

In addition to the above guidance, the RDN may recommend adjusting dietary potassium intake to maintain serum potassium within normal limits for adults with CKD 5D (OPINION).[2] The 2020 KDQOI guideline also suggests that for adults with CKD stage 5D (2D) with either hyperkalemia or hypokalemia, "dietary or supplemental potassium intake be based on a patient's individual needs and clinician judgment."[2] Hypokalemia or hyperkalemia can have a direct effect on cardiac function, with potential for cardiac arrhythmia and sudden death.[7]

Calcium

The 2020 KDOQI guideline suggests adjusting "calcium intake (dietary calcium, calcium supplements, or calcium-based binders) with consideration for concurrent use of vitamin D analogs and calcimimetics in order to avoid hypercalcemia or calcium overload (OPINION)."[2] Caution regarding elemental calcium intake is warranted, as extracellular fluid calcium levels increase with an elemental daily calcium intake above 1.5 g, with the excess extracellular calcium leading to soft tissue calcification.[2]

Hypercalcemia may contribute to nonfatal cardiovascular events and mortality.[2] When working with a patient with hypercalcemia who is on maintenance dialysis, the 2020 KDOQI guideline suggests the following[2]:

- For patients taking calcium-based phosphate binders, "the dose should be reduced or therapy switched to a noncalcium phosphate binder."
- For patients taking active vitamin D analogs, "the dose should be reduced or therapy discontinued until serum concentration of calcium returns to normal."
- "If hypercalcemia persists, consider using a low dialysate calcium concentration (1.5–2 mEq/L). This should be done with caution because observational studies have linked this approach with increased risk for arrhythmia and heart failure."[2]

Phosphorus

Hyperphosphatemia begins to appear when GFR is below 45 mL/min/1.73 m^2.[2] Because CKD-MBD is common in patients with CKD, phosphorus control is essential for the treatment and prevention of secondary hyperparathyroidism, renal bone disease, and soft tissue calcification.[7]

For adults with CKD stage 5D (1B), dietary phosphorus intake should be evaluated and adjustments to phosphorus intake are recommended to achieve serum phosphorus within normal levels.[2] The RDN should assess the patient's diet history to evaluate the bioavailability of phosphorus (see Table 4.6) from foods consumed and from phosphorus additives when developing diet recommendations (OPINION).[2]

To help decrease phosphorus intake, the 2020 KDOQI guideline suggests counseling patients to do the following[2]:

- Choose whole and/or minimally processed natural foods with low phosphorus content, and specifically a low amount of organic phosphorus per 1 g protein. Nutrient composition tables are a helpful resource.
- Avoid industry-prepared foods with phosphorus additives.
- Cook at home using wet (ie, boiling) preparation methods. Food palatability may be impacted, but up to 50% of phosphorus may be removed.

TABLE 4.6 Phosphorus Absorption From Various Diet Sources[2]

Dietary source of phosphorus	Percentage of phosphorus absorbed in the gastrointestinal tract
Animal-based foods	40%-60%
Plant-based foods	20%-50%
Phosphorus additives	Approximately 100%

The dose and timing of phosphate binders should be individually adjusted to the phosphate content of meals and snacks to achieve desired serum phosphorus levels. Serum phosphorus levels are difficult to control with dietary restrictions alone. Treatment to manage serum phosphorus needs to be individualized and may include dietary phosphate restriction, phosphate binders, calcium and vitamin D supplementation, and self-management training.[7]

Aluminum

The kidneys are involved in the excretion of aluminum, and aluminum can accumulate in the body of adults with CKD.[31] Therefore, long-term use of aluminum-containing phosphorus binders should be avoided to prevent aluminum intoxication,[9,13-15] encephalopathy, neurotoxicity, and osteomalacia.[17]

Iron

The recommended daily intake of iron is 8 mg for males and 15 mg for females.[18] When a patient receives an erythropoiesis-stimulating agent, additional supplemental oral iron is appropriate (unless the patient is receiving intravenous iron) to maintain adequate serum transferrin and serum ferritin levels and to achieve a target hemoglobin concentration of 9 to 11.5 g/dL.[16] To improve iron absorption, oral iron supplements should be taken between meals and not with phosphorus binders.[16]

Magnesium

There are currently no evidenced-based guidelines that evaluate the appropriate daily intake of magnesium in CKD. Magnesium-containing antacid medications (eg, Maalox, Phillip's Milk of Magnesia) may cause blood/serum levels of magnesium to rise in patients with CKD.[17]

Zinc

Zinc intake for adults with CKD should mirror the RDA for the general population.[2] Daily nutritional intake of 8 to 12 mg elemental zinc for females and 10 to 15 mg for males is recommended.[18] When a patient's zinc intake is chronically inadequate and the patient has symptoms of zinc deficiency (impaired taste or smell, skin fragility, impotence, or peripheral neuropathy), daily supplementation with 50 mg elemental zinc may be considered for 3 to 6 months.[18] At that time, biochemical levels should be rechecked, and zinc supplementation should be discontinued if serum levels have normalized.[18]

Zinc supplementation, in high doses or over a long period of time, may lead to copper deficiency, which, if undiagnosed, may cause irreversible neurologic conditions.[19] The 2020 KDOQI guideline does not recommend routine zinc supplementation (2C).[2] RDNs should be familiar with signs and symptoms of zinc deficiency in order to recommend and monitor supplementation when needed.

Selenium

Selenium intake for adults with CKD should mirror the RDA for the general population.[2] Daily intake of 55 mcg selenium is appropriate,[18] but the 2020 KDOQI guideline does not recommend routine selenium supplementation (2C).[2] It may be appropriate for patients on HD and with symptoms of selenium deficiency (eg, cardiomyopathy, skeletal myopathy, thyroid dysfunction, hemolysis, or dermatosis) to take selenium supplements for 3 to 6 months.[18] RDNs should be familiar with signs and symptoms of selenium deficiency in order to recommend and monitor supplementation when needed.[2]

Fluid Prescription: Chronic Kidney Disease 5D

Current fluid intake guidelines for patients on MHD vary from 500 to 750 mL/d plus urine output.[18] In general, achievement of this goal will support an interdialytic weight gain of 2 to 2.5 kg.[18]

Evidence-based guidelines have not been established for fluid intake for PD. The goal for the patient on PD should be to maintain fluid balance.

Nutritional Supplementation: Chronic Kidney Disease 5D

To develop strategies to combat PEW in patients on dialysis, the 2020 KDOQI work group[2] reviewed current research and determined guidance for ONS, enteral tube feeding, intradialytic parenteral nutrition (IDPN), and amino acid dialysate/intraperitoneal amino acid (IPAA) supplementation.

Oral Nutrition Supplements

Patients with CKD may struggle to meet recommended calorie and protein needs despite receiving regular diet counseling from a renal RDN.

The 2020 KDOQI guideline for adults with CKD stage 5D (2D) at risk of or with PEW suggests "a minimum of a 3-month trial of oral nutritional supplements to improve nutritional status if dietary counseling alone does not achieve sufficient energy and protein intake to meet nutritional requirements."[2]

Following a complete nutrition assessment, consider the following for ONS use[2]:

- Prescribe ONS two to three times per day.
- ONS should be consumed 1 hour after meals.
- Track in-center consumption of ONS toward calculated calorie and protein needs.
- Prescribe ONS that meets patient preferences such as taste, smell, texture, and appearance.
- Monitor patients for gastrointestinal symptoms when ONS is prescribed.
- ONS formulated for the renal patient "may be necessary to increase protein and energy intake and avoid fluid overload and electrolyte derangements."

Enteral Nutrition Prescription

Patients with renal failure who require nutrition support therapy should receive enteral nutrition if their intestinal function permits.[20] Macronutrient, vitamin, and mineral guidelines for CKD may apply to the enteral prescription.[21] The patient's serum concentrations of potassium, magnesium, phosphorus, and calcium should be monitored so electrolyte intake can be adjusted appropriately.[20]

The 2020 KDOQI guideline suggests that for adults with CKD stage 5D (OPINION) "with chronically inadequate intake and whose protein and energy requirements cannot be attained by dietary counseling and oral nutrition supplements, it is reasonable to consider a trial of enteral tube feeding."[2] Box 5.2 on page 136 lists a selection of available enteral formulas.

Intradialytic Parenteral Nutrition

If energy and protein needs are not being met after a trial of ONS and enteral nutrition for a patient with CKD stage 5 and PEW on MHD, the 2020 KDOQI guideline suggests a trial of intradialytic parenteral nutrition (IDPN) "... to improve and maintain nutritional status if nutritional requirements cannot be met with existing oral and enteral intake." (2C)[2]

The evidence review found no benefit to IDPN over ONS and stated that "IDPN should be considered in conjunction with ONS or dietary counseling" because IDPN can only be provided during a HD treatment, which limits the nutrition that can be delivered.[2]

When contemplating initiating IDPN, practitioners should plan for the following[2]:

- the possibility of infection, especially if the HD catheter is used to deliver the IDPN;
- the cost of IDPN therapy;
- close monitoring and evaluation of the patient nutrition parameters and adjustment of the HD prescription and medications as needed;
- IDPN should be discontinued as soon as nutrition status improves; and
- the need for PN should be evaluated if nutrition status does not improve with IDPN and ONS, or enteral nutrition is not tolerated.

The 2020 KDOQI work group indicated that patients on MHD who meet all of the following three criteria may benefit from IDPN therapy[2]:

- "evidence of PEW and inadequate dietary protein and/or energy intake";
- "inability to administer or tolerate adequate oral nutrition, including food supplements or enteral feeding"; and
- "protein and energy requirements can be met when IDPN is used in conjunction with oral intake or enteral feeding."

A more detailed discussion of IDPN administration is beyond the scope of this guide. Support for administration and monitoring of IDPN (eg, formula calculations, infusion rates, metabolic and laboratory monitors) may be available from companies that provide IDPN.[23,25] Refer to Box 4.8[23,25] for macronutrient and electrolyte considerations for IDPN.

BOX 4.8 Macronutrient and Electrolyte Considerations in Intradialytic Parenteral Nutrition[23,25]

General considerations

"The optimal intradialytic parenteral nutrition (IDPN) formulation is not known."[23]

Amino acids

IDPN formulas provide essential and nonessential amino acids (AAs).[23,25]

Standard IDPN formulas provide 1.2 to 1.4 g AA/kg body weight.[23,25] Higher protein levels can be considered in acute illness.[23]

To avoid acidosis, monitor serum bicarbonate levels and adjust to 24 to 26 mmol/L.[23]

Dextrose

Check peripheral glucose 1 hour before IDPN, at least once per hour into an infusion, and 1 hour after an infusion of IDPN.[23,25]

Consider providing a snack a half-hour before an IDPN treatment is completed to combat potential hypoglycemia.[23,25]

If blood glucose is greater than 300 mg/dL, consider 5 to 8 units of insulin per 1,000 mL IDPN.[23,25]

Increase insulin by 2 units per treatment to reach an acceptable level of blood glucose control.[23,25]

Tight glycemic control has not been studied in patients receiving IDPN but may not be appropriate due to the hazards of hypoglycemia.[23,25]

Lipids

Research has not determined whether lipids are required in IDPN.[23]

Check serum triglycerides prior to first two IDPN treatments; continue to recheck every month.[23,25]

If triglycerides are greater than 400 mg/dL, data suggest that lipids are not being well cleared.[23,25]

Avoid lipids if the patient is allergic to egg, olive oil, peanut, fish, and/or soy.[23]

Monitor for symptoms of lipid intolerance including nausea, vomiting, headache, dizziness, fever, flushing, drowsiness, muscle pain, and cramps.[23]

Electrolytes

Intracellular shifts of electrolytes can result from the glucose infusion.[25]
Monitor potassium, phosphorus, and magnesium levels at each dialysis treatment until they are stable; then check monthly.[23,25]

Amino Acid Dialysate/Intraperitoneal Amino Acid Supplementation

The 2020 KDOQI work group states that for adults with CKD stage 5D on PD and with PEW, "we suggest not substituting conventional dextrose dialysate with amino acid dialysate as a general strategy to improve nutritional status, although it is reasonable to consider a trial of amino acid dialysate to improve and maintain nutritional status if nutritional requirements cannot be met with existing oral and enteral intake (OPINION)."[2]

When contemplating initiating IPAA supplementation, practitioners should consider the following[2]:

- Treat low bicarbonate levels that may result from IPAA supplementation.
- Amino acid PD solutions may improve blood glucose control in patients with diabetes.
- "IPAA should only be used if spontaneous protein and energy intakes in conjunction with IPAA are able to meet the required protein and energy targets. Otherwise, daily [PN] or partial parenteral nutrition should be considered."

Parenteral Nutrition Prescription

When altered gastrointestinal function makes the use of the gastrointestinal tract and enteral nutrition impossible, PN may be considered. The PN prescription should be calculated based on acute and chronic medical issues using the patient's edema-free estimated dry or target weight.[23] Practitioners should take special care to accurately calculate and advance the PN prescription to avoid elevated blood glucose and electrolyte imbalances, including refeeding syndrome.[21]

The 2016 American Society for Parenteral and Enteral Nutrition guidelines for the adult critically ill patient suggest that "hypocaloric PN dosing ($\leq$20 kcal/kg/d or 80% of estimated energy needs) with adequate protein ... be considered in appropriate patients (high risk or severely malnourished) requiring PN, initially over the first week of hospitalization in the intensive care unit (ICU)."[21] The proposed benefits of this strategy include improved blood glucose control, less insulin resistance and infectious morbidity, and reduced length of intubation and hospital length of stay.[21] Caloric needs provided by PN can be calculated and adjusted to meet 100% of estimated energy requirements when the patient's condition is stable.[21] See Box 4.8.

Other Dialysis Schedules

Conventional home hemodialysis is comparable to thrice-weekly in-center hemodialysis (the most common schedule used in the United States).[32] However, when a patient is on dialysis at home, the patient's physician may prescribe more frequent dialysis, which has been shown to improve quality of life and clinical outcomes while changing nutrition considerations.[32-34]

Short daily home hemodialysis may be performed five to seven times per week for 2 to 3 hours per treatment.[32,25]

Nocturnal hemodialysis (NHD) is currently performed either at a dialysis facility with a medical team or as nocturnal home hemodialysis (NHHD) done by a patient with a care partner.[23,32] See Table 4.7 for a comparison of weekly HD treatment times between modalities.[32,35-37] NHD, including NHHD, may allow a more individualized diet (see Box 4.9 on page 112 for guidelines),[23] while considering adjustments for

TABLE 4.7 Comparison of Hemodialysis Treatment Times[32,35-37]

Hemodialysis type	Number of treatments per week	Treatment duration, hours	Total weekly treatment time, hours
In-center	3	3-4 or more	9-12 or more
In-center nocturnal	3	8	24
Conventional home	3	3-4 or more	9-12 or more
Short daily home	5-7	2-3	10-21
Nocturnal home	Every other night, up to six times per week	6-8	18-48

BOX 4.9	**Nutrition Guidelines for Nocturnal Hemodialysis Administered at Home[23]**
Energy	25 to 35 kcal/kg actual or adjusted body weight per day; adjust for weight loss/gain
Protein	1 to 1.2 g protein/kg actual or adjusted body weight per day; adjust for additional protein needs
Fat	Lower serum triglycerides may be seen; if serum lipids are increased, intake of dietary fat and cholesterol should be limited
Fluid	Restriction not necessary unless fluid intake exceeds maximum treatment fluid removal of 0.4 to 0.6 kg/h or 400 to 600 mL/h
Sodium	Amount guided by fluid and blood pressure goals; patients who are normotensive should strive for 2,300 mg/d
Potassium	Restriction rarely needed but should be considered if hyperkalemia occurs; recommend augmented potassium intake in patients with hypokalemia to limit problems such as muscle cramping
Phosphorus	Should be monitored and supplemented when serum levels are low
Vitamins	Renal multivitamin should be prescribed to replace water-soluble vitamins lost with dialysis

cultural food preferences and medical history.[25] Compared with thrice-weekly hemodialysis, the increased dialysis time of NHD, NHHD, and short daily home HD may result in a decreased need for diet and fluid restrictions and promote an improved appetite.[34] If a patient has renal laboratory values outside of goal ranges despite receiving dialysis more than thrice weekly (eg, with NHD, NHHD, or daily home HD), the RDN should explore the patient's dietary choices and advise diet adjustments as needed.[34] Research suggests that more frequent dialysis may result in improved clinical outcomes, but more studies are needed.[36]

Planning the Nutrition Prescription: Kidney Transplant

Care of the transplant patient is divided into three categories: pretransplantation, acute post transplantation, and chronic post transplantation.[23]

Pretransplantation Medical Nutrition Therapy

Prior to transplantation, a full evaluation of the patient's nutrition status should be completed to establish nutrition needs, determine education needed on pretransplantation and posttransplantation nutrition, and achieve ideal weight per transplant facility guidelines.[23] To establish the optimal nutrition prescription prior to kidney transplantation, the RDN should align the stage of kidney disease with the appropriate CKD nutrition evidence-based practice guidelines.[23] A more in-depth review of pretransplantation nutrition care is beyond the scope of this pocket guide.

Acute and Chronic Posttransplantation Medical Nutrition Therapy

Box 4.10[7,9,10,23,38] on page 114 and Box 4.11[2,7,9,23,38] on page 115 and the following sections review acute and chronic MNT recommendations for the patient after kidney transplant. Posttransplantation dietary recommendations are based on allograph function.

Dietary Patterns: Post Transplantation

The 2020 KDOQI guideline evaluates the benefits of following various dietary patterns for adults with CKD.[2] The work group concluded that for adults post transplantation with or without dyslipidemia, "we

BOX 4.10 Acute-Phase[a] Medical Nutrition Therapy After Kidney Transplant[7,9,10,23,38]

Energy[b,10,23,38]	Basal energy expenditure × 1.3 to 1.5
	30 to 35 kcal/kg weight
Protein[b,23,38]	1.3 to 2 g/kg weight with functioning allograft
Carbohydrate	Promote intake of complex carbohydrates[23]
	Carbohydrate-controlled diet for blood glucose control, as needed[23,38]
Fat[23]	Promote intake of heart-healthy fats
Fluid	Ad libitum[23,38]
	Adjust to graft function[23]
Vitamins	Dietary Reference Intakes (DRIs)[23]
	Supplementation is usually not necessary[38]
Minerals	
Sodium	Unrestricted if hypertension and edema are absent[23,38]; initiate restriction if hypertension or edema occur[10]
Potassium	Unrestricted unless patient has hyperkalemia[38]; if patient has hyperkalemia, less than 2.4 g/d[7]
Calcium	1,200 to 1,500 mg/d[23]; supplement if necessary[38]; measure weekly until stable[9]
Phosphorus	DRI[23]; supplement if necessary[38]; measure weekly until stable[9]
Magnesium	DRI[23]; supplement if necessary[38]

[a] Acute phase = 8 weeks immediately post transplant.
[b] Based on standard or adjusted body weight.

BOX 4.11 Chronic-Phase Medical Nutrition Therapy After Kidney Transplant[2,7,9,23,38]

Energy	25 to 35 kcal/kg/d (OPINION) to maintain normal nutritional status[2]
	Achieve desirable body weight[2,23,38]
	Adjust for weight goals, age, sex, physical activity, body composition, stage of chronic kidney disease (CKD), and metabolic stressors[2,7]
Protein	0.8 to 1 g/kg/d with functioning allograft[7,23,38]; insufficient evidence to recommend plant vs animal protein (OPINION)[2]
Carbohydrate	Promote intake of complex carbohydrates[23]
	Carbohydrate-controlled diet for blood glucose control, as needed[23,38]
Fat	Promote intake of heart-healthy fats[23]
	Long-chain omega-3 polyunsaturated fatty acids; no routine supplementation recommended to lower risk of mortality (2C) or cardiovascular events (2B) or to reduce the number of rejection episodes or improve graft survival (2D).[2]
Fluid	Ad libitum[38]
Micronutrients	Encourage oral intake that provides the Recommended Dietary Allowances for vitamins and minerals (OPINION)[2]
Multivitamin (MVI) supplement	Evaluate oral intake and consider MVI supplement when intake is inadequate (OPINION)[2]

Continued on next page

BOX 4.11 Chronic-Phase Medical Nutrition Therapy After Kidney Transplant (cont.)[2,7,9,23,38]

Vitamins	Dietary Reference Intakes (DRI)[23]; supplement as needed[38]
Folate/ vitamin B12/ B-complex	With deficiency/insufficiency, suggest folate, vitamin B12, and/or B-complex supplement (OPINION)[2]; no routine supplementation with the diagnosis of hyperhomocysteinemia, to reduce adverse cardiovascular outcomes (1A)[2]
Vitamin C	At least 90 mg/d for males and 75 mg/d for females (OPINION) at risk of deficiency[2]
Vitamin D	With deficiency/insufficiency, suggest supplementation with cholecalciferol or ergocalciferol (OPINION)[2]; treat deficiency/insufficiency using treatment strategies for the general population[9]
Vitamin K	Avoid vitamin K supplements in patients taking anticoagulant medications (eg, warfarin compounds) (OPINION)[2]

Minerals/Electrolytes

Sodium	Less than 2.3 g/d (1C) to control blood pressure and volume status[2]
Potassium	To keep potassium within normal limits, evaluate individual needs and use clinical judgment to recommend dietary supplementation or restriction as needed (OPINION)[2]; if patient has hyperkalemia, less than 2.4 g/d[7]
Calcium	1,200 to 1,500 mg/d[23]; not to exceed 2,000 mg/d from all sources[7]
Phosphorus	DRI[23]; evaluate bioavailability of dietary phosphorus (eg, animal, vegetable, additives) when considering phosphorus restriction (OPINION)[2]; replete hypophosphatemia with diet or a supplement when patient has CKD post transplantation (OPINION)[2,7]
Magnesium	DRI[23]; supplement or restrict as needed[38]

suggest that prescribing a Mediterranean Diet may improve lipid profiles (2C)."[2] The RDN should use clinical judgment to evaluate whether the Mediterranean diet is appropriate for the individual patient based on the function of the allograph and serum potassium levels.[2]

Protein Prescription: Post Transplantation

In the acute posttransplantation phase, defined as the first 4 to 8 weeks after the transplant, the patient should consume between 1.3 and 2 g of protein per kilogram per day to reverse negative nitrogen balance and boost muscle mass.[23,38]

After surgical recovery during the chronic posttransplantation phase, defined as greater than 8 weeks post transplantation, adult kidney transplant recipients with an adequately functioning transplanted kidney or allograft should consume 0.8 to 1 g of protein per kilogram per day.[7,23,38] Adequate, but not excessive, protein intake supports allograft survival and minimizes the risk of comorbid conditions.[7]

The 2020 KDOQI work group reviewed the research to evaluate whether there is a benefit to consuming animal or vegetable protein diets on nutritional status, CKD-MBD, or lipid levels.[2] The work group concluded that there was not enough evidence to promote consumption of animal or plant protein in adults post transplantation, for the stated areas of interest (OPINION).[2]

Energy Prescription: Post Transplantation

It is important to use clinical judgment to determine the ideal edema-free body weight to use for energy calculations for patients after a kidney transplant.[7] Energy needs in the first 8 weeks after transplant are typically 30 to 35 kcal/kg/d.[23,38] However, energy requirements during this time period may be higher when there are postoperative complications.[23]

For the chronic posttransplant patient who is metabolically stable, energy intake is recommended at 25 and 35 kcal/kg/d.[2] Refer to Box 4.2 for an overview of the term metabolically stable.[2] Maintenance of a desirable weight is an appropriate goal.[23,38]

Carbohydrate Prescription: Post Transplantation

For adults post transplant with a diagnosis of diabetes, the RDN should follow published evidence-based guidelines for the treatment of diabetes[23] and implement MNT recommendations to achieve a target HbA1c of approximately 7%.[7] Intensive treatment of hyperglycemia while avoiding hypoglycemia prevents complications, such as retinopathy and neuropathy, and may slow the progression of established kidney disease. If the patient develops new-onset diabetes after transplantation, dietary carbohydrate should be prescribed as recommended for the care of patients with diabetes.[7]

Fat Prescription: Post Transplantation

Cardiovascular disease is the leading cause of death post transplantation.[23] The fat prescription should set healthful targets for the amounts and types of fat consumed (eg, saturated, *trans*, polyunsaturated, and monounsaturated), with goal of improving lipid parameters (see Boxes 4.10 and 4.11).

The 2020 KDOQI work group assessed the benefits of long-chain omega-3 PUFA for the posttransplantation population and developed the following recommendations[2]:

- For adults who are post transplant, "we suggest not routinely prescribing long-chain omega-3 PUFA, including those derived from fish or flaxseed and other oils, to lower risk of mortality (2C) or cardiovascular events (2B)."
- For adults with CKD after transplantation, "we suggest not routinely prescribing long-chain omega-3 PUFA to reduce the number of rejection episodes or improve graft survival (2D)."

Micronutrient Prescription: Post Transplantation

The 2020 KDOQI work group reviewed the research regarding micronutrient needs of the patient post transplant and provided the following expert opinions and recommendations for vitamin and mineral intake for adults post transplantation[2]:

- "[I]t is reasonable for the registered dietitian nutritionist (RDN) or international equivalent to encourage eating a diet that meets the recommended dietary allowance (RDA) for adequate intake for all vitamins and minerals (OPINION)."
- "[I]t is reasonable for the registered dietitian nutritionist (RDN) or international equivalent, in close collaboration with a physician or physician assistant, to assess dietary vitamin intake periodically and to consider multivitamin supplementation for individuals with inadequate vitamin intake (OPINION)."

Vitamin Prescription: Post Transplantation

See Boxes 4.10 and 4.11 for vitamin recommendations for the patient who is post–kidney transplant, in addition to the following recommendations:

- For adults post transplantation (OPINION), "we suggest prescribing **vitamin D** supplementation in the form of cholecalciferol or ergocalciferol to correct 25-hydroxyvitamin D (25(OH)D) deficiency/insufficiency."[3] Sufficient vitamin D should be recommended to maintain levels of serum 25-hydroxyvitamin D equal to or greater than 30 ng/mL.[7]
- For adults post transplantation and who are "at risk of **vitamin C** deficiency, it is reasonable to consider supplementation to meet the recommended intake of at least 90 mg/d for men and 75 mg/d for women (OPINION)."[2] Vitamin C supplementation is sometimes used to improve iron absorption for patients post transplantation who have iron-deficiency anemia. There is insufficient evidence to recommend vitamin C supplementation greater than the DRI in the management of iron-deficiency anemia, because supplemental vitamin C can increase the risk of hyperoxalosis.[7]
- For adults post transplantation, "it is reasonable that patients receiving anticoagulant medicines known to inhibit **vitamin K** activity (eg, warfarin compounds) do not receive vitamin K supplements (OPINION)."[2]

- For adults post transplantation and "who have hyperhomocysteinemia associated with kidney disease, we recommend not to routinely supplement **folate** with or without B-complex since there is no evidence demonstrating reduction in adverse cardiovascular outcomes (1A)."[2]
- For adults post transplantation (OPINION), "we suggest prescribing **folate**, vitamin B12, and/or B-complex supplement to correct for folate or vitamin B12 deficiency/insufficiency based on clinical signs and symptoms."[2]

When a posttransplant patient is assessed to be at higher nutritional risk due to poor dietary intake and decreasing GFR, a multivitamin preparation should be recommended.[7]

Electrolyte and Mineral Prescription: Post Transplantation

Boxes 4.10 and 4.11 list electrolyte and mineral recommendations for the patient who is post–kidney transplant. Additional recommendations are as follows.

Sodium

During the acute posttransplantation period, with adequate allograph function, sodium recommendations should mirror the intake for the general population.[10]

The 2020 KDOQI guideline states that for adults post transplantation (1C), "we recommend limiting sodium intake to less than 100 mmol/d (or <2.3 g/d) to reduce blood pressure and improve volume control."[2] This target should be adjusted as appropriate based on fluid balance, blood pressure control, and other clinical findings.[2,7] Some resources suggest that dietary sodium intake can safely range from 2 to 4 g/d after a kidney transplant.[23,38]

Potassium

A kidney transplant generally leads to normalized serum potassium levels; in which case, dietary potassium restriction is not necessary.[23]

However, elevated serum potassium levels may be caused by a poorly functioning graft or adverse effects of medications such as calcineurin inhibitors.[23] When a patient who has had a kidney transplant has hyperkalemia, a potassium intake of less than 2.4 g/d should be recommended, with consideration of other clinical factors, including serum potassium levels, medications that may affect potassium levels, glycemic control, and other issues.[7]

Hypokalemia has also been reported in kidney transplant recipients and may be caused by potassium-wasting diuretics.[23] Hypokalemia or hyperkalemia can have direct effects on cardiac function, with a potential for cardiac arrhythmia and sudden death.[7]

The 2020 KDOQI guideline states the following[2]:

- For adults post transplantation (OPINION) "with either hyperkalemia or hypokalemia, we suggest that dietary or supplemental potassium intake be based on a patient's individual needs and clinical judgment."
- For adults post transplantation, "it is reasonable to adjust dietary potassium intake to maintain serum potassium within the normal range (OPINION)."

Calcium

During the acute phase of kidney transplantation, calcium supplementation should be limited to 1,200 to 1,500 mg/d.[23]

For the chronic phase of kidney transplantation, the RDN should recommend a calcium intake (including dietary calcium, calcium supplementation, and calcium-based phosphate binders) of 2,000 mg/d or less.[7] Patients with CKD are predisposed to mineral and bone disorders. Serum calcium concentration is an important factor in regulating PTH secretion, which affects bone integrity and soft tissue calcification.[7] The RDN should be aware of the risks of hypercalcemia, including soft tissue calcification.[7]

Phosphorus

Hypophosphatemia is most common in the early weeks after a kidney transplant.[7] For adult kidney transplant recipients with low serum phosphorus, the RDN should recommend or prescribe a high-phosphorus diet or supplements containing phosphorus (see Box 5.1 on page 134) to replete serum phosphorus as needed.[7] Generally, the DRI for phosphorus is appropriate for patients post–kidney transplant.[23]

The 2020 KDOQI guideline states the following[2]:

- For adults post transplantation, "it is reasonable when making decisions about phosphorus restriction treatment to consider the bioavailability of phosphorus sources (eg, animal, vegetable, additives) (OPINION)."

- For adults with CKD post transplantation with hypophosphatemia, "it is reasonable to consider prescribing high-phosphorus intake (diet or supplement) in order to replete serum phosphate (OPINION)."

Iron

Anemia guidelines from Kidney Disease Improving Global Outcomes (KDIGO) in 2012 updated ferritin and TSAT cutoffs for patients with CKD, but not for transplant patients specifically.[16] According to the Academy of Nutrition and Dietetics Evidence Analysis Library CKD recommendations, when a patient's serum ferritin level is equal to or less than 100 ng/mL post transplant and TSAT is equal to or less than 20%, oral or intravenous iron supplementation may be recommended.[7] The amount of iron supplementation recommended should maintain levels of serum iron that will adequately support erythropoiesis. Iron absorption may be impaired by other medications, such as phosphate binders.[7]

Nutritional Supplementation: Post Transplantation

To develop strategies to combat PEW in patients post transplantation, the 2020 KDOQI work group reviewed current research and determined guidance for ONS.[2]

Oral Nutrition Supplements

Patients may struggle to meet recommended calorie and protein needs post transplant despite receiving regular diet counseling from a renal RDN.[2] The 2020 KDOQI guideline recommends that for adults post transplantation (OPINION) at risk of or with PEW, "we suggest a minimum of a 3-month trial of oral nutritional supplements to improve nutritional status if dietary counseling alone does not achieve sufficient energy and protein intake to meet nutritional requirements."[2]

Enteral and Parenteral Nutrition Prescription

If enteral nutrition or PN is necessary after a kidney transplant, refer to the evidence-based guidelines that dictate the appropriate MNT based on the function of the allograph.

Case Study

Nutrition Care Process

Step 3: Nutrition Intervention

Part 1: Planning the Nutrition Prescription

> This chapter adds the first part of the nutrition intervention piece of the NCP to information captured in the assessment presented in Chapter 2 and development of the diagnosis presented in Chapter 3. New information is set off from the previous material in white. This section presents the steps followed in planning the patient's nutrition prescription. Later chapters continue to develop the case with information appropriate to each step of the NCP.

A 56-year-old female individual with CKD stage 5D on peritoneal dialysis is admitted to the hospital.

Nutrition Assessment

Food/Nutrition-Related History

Food Intake
Patient consumes traditional Cambodian foods and follows traditional Cambodian meal patterns, including rice, stir-fried vegetables, and small amounts of fish, poultry, and beef. Uses fish sauce frequently. Has been consuming increased amounts of cola soft drinks to ease nausea.

Medications
HMG-CoA reductase inhibitor (statin), renal multivitamin, calcium carbonate and sevelamer with meals, calcitriol, ferrous sulfate, insulin aspart with meals, isoniazid, vitamin B6, and lansoprazole. Has missed a few days of taking medications because of current condition.

Food and Nutrition Knowledge/Skill
Family is aware of low phosphorus and low potassium foods; is very involved.

Physical activity
Sedentary

Anthropometric Measurements

Body Composition, Growth, and Weight History
Height
150 cm (59 in)

Admit weight
74.5 kg (164 lb)

Estimated dry weight (EDW)
72 kg (has been stable)

BMI (using EDW)
32

Frame size
Medium

Ideal body weight (IBW)
62 kg; 116% IBW

Biochemical Data, Medical Tests, and Procedures

Electrolyte and renal profile
See laboratory data table.

Nutritional anemia profile
See laboratory data table.

Urine output
500 mL/24 h

Laboratory Data for Nutrition Assessment of Patient[3]

Laboratory test	Reference range	Patient result
Potassium, mmol/L	Normal: 3.4-5 Peritoneal dialysis (PD)[a]: 3.5-5.5	5.4
Blood urea nitrogen, mg/dL	Normal: 6-20 PD: >60	58
Creatinine, mg/dL	Normal: 0.7-1.3 PD: not defined	11
Glucose, mg/dL	Normal (fasting): 60-99	92
Calcium, mg/dL	Normal: 8.6-10.2	8.8
Phosphorus, mg/dL	Normal: 2.4-4.7 PD: 3.5-5.5	5.7

Continued on next page

Laboratory Data for Nutrition Assessment of Patient (cont.)[a]

Laboratory test	Reference range	Patient result
Albumin, g/dL	Normal: 3.5-4.7 PD: >3.5	1.6
Hemoglobin, g/dL	Normal: 13.5-17.5 PD: 10-12	9
Capillary blood glucose, mg/dL	Normal: <150	120-250
Sodium, mmol/L	Normal: 134-143	129

[a] Reference range for patients on peritoneal dialysis.

Nutrition Focused Physical Findings

- Overall appearance: abrasions on arms and neck from scratching
- Obese with central adiposity
- Bilateral ankle edema and edema of eyelid
- Diarrhea, nausea, and vomiting
- Pale conjunctiva
- Koilonychia (spoon-shaped nails)

Patient History

Personal data: Patient is 56-year-old female individual, does not speak English; children are fluent in English and are very involved and supportive.

Patient or family nutrition-oriented medical/health history: ESRD due to hypertension. History includes type 2 diabetes. Admitted to the hospital with peritonitis, pain, nausea, vomiting, and fever. Third episode of peritonitis in 2 months. Latent tuberculosis.

Treatment/therapy: Peritoneal dialysis with five exchanges per day, each 2 L 2.5% dextrose. Type 2 diabetes mellitus managed with insulin; capillary blood glucose usually less than 250 mg/dL.

Nutrition Diagnosis

Intake Domain

Nutrition Diagnosis
Excessive mineral intake (sodium)

Sample PES Statement
Excessive sodium intake related to cultural food patterns as evidenced by diet recall revealing frequent use of fish sauce as well as presence of ankle and orbital edema.

Clinical Domain

Nutrition Diagnosis
Altered nutrition-related laboratory values (serum phosphorus and albumin)

Sample PES Statements
- Altered nutrition-related laboratory values (serum phosphorus) related to missed binder doses as evidenced by patient report and serum phosphorus value of 5.7 mg/dL.
- Altered nutrition-related laboratory values (serum albumin) related to altered nutrient utilization in inflammatory state as evidenced by serum albumin of 1.6 g/dL in a patient with acute peritonitis.

Behavioral-Environmental Domain

Nutrition Diagnosis
Limited adherence to nutrition-related recommendations

Sample PES Statement

Limited adherence to nutrition-related recommendations related to the use of high-phosphorus soft drinks to treat gastrointestinal symptoms as evidenced by patient reports of drinking cola beverages during episodes of nausea.

Nutrition Intervention

Peritoneal Dialysis Regimen

Patient receives PD with five exchanges per day, each 2 L 2.5% dextrose.

Note: 2.5% dextrose provides 25 g dextrose/L (see Table 4.7 for additional information on dextrose contributions).

Calculate calories from daily PD exchanges as follows:

2 L per exchange × (25 g dextrose/L) = 50 g dextrose per PD exchange

(50 g dextrose per PD exchange) × (5 PD exchanges/d) = 250 g dextrose/d

(250 g dextrose/d) × (3.4 kcal/g dextrose) = 850 kcal/d

(850 kcal/d) × 70% absorption = 595 kcal/d from PD exchanges

Calculating Energy and Protein Needs

Note: Calculation uses dry weight
Energy needs:

72 kg × 25 to 30 kcal/kg/d = 1,800 to 2,160 kcal/d

Subtract 595 kcal provided by PD regimen = 1,205 to 1,565 kcal/d

Protein needs (increased due to peritonitis):

72 kg × 1.3 g/kg/d = 94 g/d

Daily Nutrition Prescription for Patient Undergoing Peritoneal Dialysis

Other elements of the nutrition prescription are as follows:

- Based on the patient's past medical history and calculated macronutrient and micronutrient needs, suggest a renal, carbohydrate-controlled diet adjusted to cultural food preferences as permissible within renal and diabetic requirements.
- Based on urine output of 500 mL/24 h and edema/hyponatremia, suggest limiting dietary fluid intake to 1,000 mL/d.
- Based on edema/hyponatremia, suggest limiting dietary sodium to approximately 2.3 g/d.
- Based on hyperphosphatemia, adjust dietary phosphorus intake, including phosphorus additives, to reduce phosphorus within normal range. Confirm patient is taking phosphorus binders with meals.
- To prevent undesirable weight gain while maintaining dry weight, limit dietary calories to approximately 1,600 kcal/d. (Patient will receive an additional 595 kcal/d from PD exchanges.)
- To replete protein stores in the context of peritonitis, provide approximately 94 g protein per day. Reevaluate adequacy of estimated protein needs at nutrition follow-up.

References

1. Academy of Nutrition and Dietetics. Electronic Nutrition Care Process Terminology (eNCPT). Accessed November 29, 2022. www.ncpro.org

2. Ikizler TA, Burrowes JD, Byham-Gray LD, et al. KDOQI clinical practice guideline for nutrition in CKD: 2020 update. *J Kidney Dis*. 2020;76(3 suppl 1):S1-S107. doi:10.1053/j.ajkd.2020.05.006

3. Kidney Disease Outcomes Quality Initiative . KDOQI clinical practice guidelines and clinical practice recommendations for diabetes and chronic kidney disease. *Am J Kidney Dis*. 2007;49(2 suppl 2):S12-S154. doi:10.1053/j.ajkd.2006.12.005

4. Kidney Disease Improving Global Outcomes. KDIGO clinical practice guideline for diabetes management in chronic kidney disease. *Kidney Int Suppl*. 2020;98(4S):S1-S115.

5. Kidney Disease Outcomes Quality Initiative (K/DOQI) Group. K/DOQI clinical practice guidelines for management of dyslipidemias in patients with kidney disease. *Am J Kidney Dis*. 2003;41(4 suppl 3):I-S91.

6. American Heart Association. *Trans* fats. American Heart Association website. March 2017. Accessed May 21, 2021. https://cpr.heart.org/en/healthy-living/healthy-eating/eat-smart/fats/trans-fat

7. Academy of Nutrition and Dietetics Evidence Analysis Library. Chronic kidney disease (CKD) guideline. 2010. Accessed August 11, 2022. www.andeal.org/topic.cfm?cat=3927&highlight=kidney&home=1

8. Kidney Disease Improving Global Outcomes (KDIGO) Blood Pressure Work Group. KDIGO 2021 clinical practice guideline for the management of blood pressure in chronic kidney disease. *Kidney Int*. 2021;99(3 suppl):S1-S87. doi:10.1016/j.kint.2020.11.003

9. Kidney Disease Improving Global Outcomes (KDIGO) CKD-MBD Update Work Group. KDIGO 2017 clinical practice guideline update for the diagnosis, evaluation, prevention, and treatment of chronic kidney disease–mineral and bone disorder (CKD-MBD). *Kidney Int Suppl*. 2017;7(1):1-59. doi:10.1016/j.kisu.2017.04.001

10. McCann L. *Pocket Guide to Nutrition Assessment of the Patient with Kidney Disease*. 6th ed. National Kidney Foundation; 2021.

11. Steiber AL, Kopple JD. Vitamin status and needs for people with stages 3-5 chronic kidney disease. *J Ren Nutr*. 2011;21(5):355-368. doi:10.1053/j.jrn.2010.12.004

12. Dawson-Hughes B. Patient education: vitamin D deficiency (beyond the basics). UpToDate website. 2023. Accessed August 31, 2023. www.uptodate.com/contents/vitamin-d-deficiency-beyond-the-basics

13. Kidney Disease Improving Global Outcomes (KDIGO) CKD-MBD Work Group. KDIGO clinical practice guideline for the diagnosis, evaluation, prevention, and treatment of chronic kidney disease–mineral and bone disorder (CKD-MBD). *Kidney Int Suppl*. 2009;(113):S1-S130. doi:10.1038/ki.2009.188

14. Isakova T, Nickolas TL, Denburg M, et al. KDOQI US commentary on the 2017 KDIGO clinical practice guideline update for the diagnosis, evaluation, prevention, and treatment of chronic kidney disease–mineral and bone disorder (CKD-MBD). *Am J Kidney Dis.* 2017;70(6):737-751. doi:10.1053/j.ajkd.2017.07.019

15. Uhlig K, Berns JS, Kestenbaum B, et al. KDOQI US commentary on the 2009 KDIGO clinical practice guideline for the diagnosis, evaluation, and treatment of CKD–mineral and bone disorder (CKD-MBD). *Am J Kidney Dis.* 2010;55(5):773-799. doi:10.1053/j.ajkd.2010.02.340

16. Kidney Disease Improving Global Outcomes. KDIGO clinical practice guideline for anemia in chronic kidney disease. *Kidney Int Suppl.* 2012;2(4):279-335. https://kdigo.org/wp-content/uploads/2016/10/KDIGO-2012-Anemia-Guideline-English.pdf

17. Pronsky ZM, Elbe D, Ayoob K, Crowe JP, Epstein S, Roberts WH. *Food and Medication Interactions*. 18th ed. Food-Medication Interactions; 2015.

18. Fouque D, Vennegoor M, ter Wee P, et al. EBPG guideline on nutrition. *Nephrol Dial Transplant*. 2007;22(suppl 2):ii45-ii87. doi:10.1093/ndt/gfm020

19. Duncan A, Yacoubian C, Watson N, Morrison I. The risk of copper deficiency in patients prescribed zinc supplements. *J Clin Pathol.* 2015;68(9):723-725. doi:10.1136/jclinpath-2014-202837

20. Brown RO, Compher C; American Society for Parenteral and Enteral Nutrition Board of Directors. A.S.P.E.N. clinical guidelines: nutrition support in adult acute and chronic renal failure. *JPEN J Parenter Enteral Nutr.* 2010;34(4):366-377. doi:10.1177/0148607110374577

21. McClave SA, Taylor BE, Martindale RG, et al. Guidelines for the provision and assessment of nutrition support therapy in the adult critically ill patient: Society of Critical Care Medicine (SCCM) and American Society for Parenteral and Enteral Nutrition (A.S.P.E.N.) *JPEN J Parenter Enteral Nutr.* 2016;40(2):159-211. doi:10.1177/0148607115621863

22. Academy of Nutrition and Dietetics. Parenteral nutrition: Parenteral formula. Nutrition Care Manual. Accessed September 3, 2021. www.nutritioncaremanual.org/topic.cfm?lvl=255693&lv3=272590&ncm_category_id=1&ncm_toc_id=272590&ncm_heading=Nutrition%20Care&lv2=255697

23. Phillips S, Gonyea J, eds. *A Clinical Guide to Nutrition Care in Kidney Disease*. 3rd ed. Academy of Nutrition and Dietetics; 2022.

24. Kidney Disease Outcomes Quality Initiative, National Kidney Foundation. Clinical practice guidelines for nutrition in chronic renal failure. *Am J Kidney Dis.* 2000;35(6 suppl 2):S17-S104. doi:10.1053/ajkd.2000.v35.aajkd03517

25. Byham-Gray L, Wiesen K, Stover J. *A Clinical Guide to Nutrition Care in Kidney Disease*. 2nd ed. Academy of Nutrition and Dietetics; 2013.

26. White JV, Guenter P, Jensen G, et al. Consensus statement of the Academy of Nutrition and Dietetics/American Society for Parenteral and Enteral Nutrition: characteristics recommended for the identification and documentation of adult malnutrition (undernutrition). *J Acad Nutr Diet.* 2012;112(5):730-738. doi:10.1016/j.jand.2012.03.012

27. Ishibe S, Peixoto AJ. Methods of assessment of volume status and intercompartmental fluid shifts in hemodialysis patients: implications in clinical practice. *Semin Dial.* 2004;17(1):37-43. doi:10.1111/j.1525-139x.2004.17112.x

28. Sinha AD, Light RP, Agarwal R. Relative plasma volume monitoring during hemodialysis aids the assessment of dry weight. *Hypertension.* 2010;55(2):305-311. doi:10.1161/HYPERTENSIONAHA.109.143974

29. McCann L, ed. *Pocket Guide to Nutrition Assessment of the Patient with Chronic Kidney Disease.* 5th ed. National Kidney Foundation: 2015.

30. Kidney Disease Improving Global Outcomes. KDIGO clinical practice guidelines for lipid management in chronic kidney disease. *Kidney Int Suppl.* 2013;3(3):259-305. https://kdigo.org/wp-content/uploads/2017/02/KDIGO-2013-Lipids-Guideline-English.pdf

31. National Kidney Foundation. K/DOQI clinical practice guidelines for bone metabolism and disease in chronic kidney disease. *Am J Kidney Dis.* 2003;42(4 suppl 3):S1-S201.

32. National Kidney Foundation. Home hemodialysis. 2015. National Kidney Foundation website. Accessed November 30, 2021. www.kidney.org/atoz/content/homehemo

33. Tomori K, Okada H. Home hemodialysis: benefits, risks, and barriers. *Contrib Nephrol.* 2018;196:178-183. doi:10.1159/000485719

34. Sikkes ME, Kooistra MP, Weijs PJ. Improved nutrition after conversion to nocturnal home hemodialysis. *J Ren Nutr.* 2009;19(6):494-499. doi:10.1053/j.jrn.2009.05.006

35. Fresenius Kidney Care. Treatment to fit your lifestyle: home hemodialysis schedules. Fresenius Kidney Care website. Accessed December 1, 2021. www.freseniuskidneycare.com/treatment/home-hemodialysis/what-to-expect

36. National Kidney Foundation. KDOQI clinical practice guideline for hemodialysis adequacy: 2015 update. *J Kidney Dis.* 2015;66(5):884-930. doi:10.1053/j.ajkd.2015.07.015

37. Davita Kidney Care. In-center hemodialysis: dialysis care day or night. Davita Kidney Care website. Accessed December 1, 2021. www.davita.com/treatment-services/dialysis/in-center-hemodialysis?p=1

38. Blue LS. Adult kidney transplantation. In: Hasse JM, Blue LS. *Comprehensive Guide to Transplant Nutrition.* American Dietetic Association; 2002:45-56.

CHAPTER 5

Nutrition Intervention—Part 2: Implementation

This chapter builds on the nutrition prescription created in Chapter 4 and offers suggestions for implementing nutrition interventions in four intervention domains for patients with chronic kidney disease (CKD)[1]:

- food and/or nutrient delivery
- nutrition education
- nutrition counseling
- coordination of nutrition care

Food and/or Nutrient Delivery

The domain of food and/or nutrient delivery is described as an individualized approach for food/nutrient provision, including meals and snacks, enteral nutrition, parenteral nutrition/intravenous fluids, nutrition supplement therapy, medical food supplement therapy, bioactive substance management, feeding assistance, management of the feeding environment, and nutrition-related medication management.[2] This intervention domain can occur in many settings, including acute and chronic care, public health and other community settings, wellness programs, and policy development for all age groups.[1,2] Categories in this domain that are frequently used in CKD management include nutritional supplement therapy (eg, vitamin and mineral supplements), medical food supplement therapy (eg, oral nutrition supplements), and nutrition-related medication management (eg, adjustment of phosphorus binders according to scope of practice/organization policy, or recommendations for phosphorus supplements as appropriate for posttransplant patients). See Box 5.1 for information on phosphorus supplementation.

BOX 5.1 Phosphorus Supplementation[a]

Phos-NaK Powder[b]

Product description	Over-the-counter; 1.5-g packets
Electrolyte content per packet	250 mg phosphorus, 160 mg sodium, and 280 mg potassium
Special instructions	Open packet and mix powder with 2.5 oz (75 mL) water or other liquid such as juice. Stir mixture well and drink.

K-Phos Original Dissolvable Tablets[c]

Product description	Prescription; tablets in 100- and 500-count bottles
Electrolyte content per tablet	14 mg phosphorus and 144 mg potassium
Special instructions	Add tablet to 6 to 8 oz (180–240 mL) water. Let tablets dissolve completely (this takes a few minutes), then stir and drink.

K-Phos MF[c]

Product description	Prescription; tablets in 100-count bottle
Electrolyte content per tablet	250 mg phosphorus, 88 mg potassium and 134 mg sodium

BOX 5.1 Phosphorus Supplementation (cont.)[a]

K-Phos No. 2[c]

Product description	Prescription; tablets in 100-count bottle
Electrolyte content per tablet	250 mg phosphorus, 88 mg potassium and 134 mg sodium

K-Phos Neutral[c]

Product description	Prescription; tablets in 100- and 500-count bottles
Electrolyte content per tablet	250 mg phosphorus, 45 mg potassium and 298 mg sodium

Phospha 250 Neutral[d]

Product description	Prescription; tablets in 100-count bottle
Electrolyte content per tablet	250 mg phosphorus, 45 mg potassium and 298 mg sodium

[a] Manufacturers may change product formulations and offerings. Check product labels and websites for current information.
[b] Manufactured by Cypress Pharmaceuticals, Madison, MS 39130.
[c] Manufactured by Beach Pharmaceuticals, Tampa, FL 33681.
[d] Manufactured by Rising Pharmaceuticals, Allendale, NJ 07401.

Additionally important in CKD are the categories of enteral nutrition and parenteral nutrition/intravenous fluids. Chapter 4 contains information on parenteral nutrition prescriptions that might be used in kidney disease. See Box 5.2 on page 136 for information on oral supplement and enteral formula products. Product information and nutrition ingredients are subject to change, and the manufacturers' websites should be consulted for the most current ingredients and nutrition analysis data.

BOX 5.2 Oral Supplements and Enteral Formulas for Chronic Kidney Disease[a]

Protein modulars

Example	Beneprotein[b]
Characteristics	100% high-quality whey protein
Indications	Inability to meet estimated protein requirements

Energy, other modulars

Example	Medium-chain triglyceride (MCT) oil[b]
Characteristics	Contains MCTs (more readily hydrolyzed and absorbed fat source)
Indications	Used when dietary fat is not well absorbed

Oral nutrition supplements—liquid and nonliquid (bar)

Example	Milkshakes, Carnation Breakfast Essentials,[b] Ensure,[c] Nutren,[b] Boost,[b] Pure Protein Bars, and ZonePerfect Bars[c]
Characteristics	Flavored for oral consumption; may contain milk
	Most liquid supplements contain 1 kcal/mL and moderate protein levels
Indications	Inability to meet requirements via diet alone
	Depending on level of kidney function and recommended use, micronutrient content should be evaluated closely

Standard enteral formulas

Example	Nutren 1.0,[b] Osmolite,[c] and Isosource[b]
Characteristics	1 kcal/mL, moderate protein content; most meet Dietary Reference Intakes for nutrients in less than 1,500 mL

BOX 5.2 Oral Supplements and Enteral Formulas for Chronic Kidney Disease (cont.)[a]

Indications	Most patients requiring enteral feeding
	Depending on level of kidney function and recommended use, micronutrient content should be evaluated closely

Fluid-restricted formulas

Example	Nutren 2.0,[b] TwoCal HN,[c] and Boost Plus[b]
Characteristics	1.5 to 2 kcal/mL, moderate protein content
Indications	Used in patients with fluid restriction
	Depending on level of kidney function and recommended use, micronutrient content should be evaluated closely

Fiber-containing formulas

Example	Jevity[c] and Nutren with Fiber[b]
Characteristics	Generally 1 kcal/mL, moderate protein
	Type and amount of fiber may vary
Indications	May help normalize bowel function in some patients
	Depending on level of kidney function and recommended use, micronutrient content should be evaluated closely

Elemental and peptide-based formulas

Example	Vivonex,[b] Peptamen,[b] Vital[c]
Characteristics	1 kcal/mL, moderate protein content. Protein source and type may vary.
Indications	Used for patients with malabsorption and extreme gastrointestinal dysfunction
	Generally unpalatable, but may be used orally in some patients

Continued on next page

> **BOX 5.2   Oral Supplements and Enteral Formulas for Chronic Kidney Disease (cont.)[a]**
>
> ***Formulas for glucose intolerance***
>
> Example — Glucerna[c]
>
> Characteristics — Usually 1 kcal/mL but can vary; moderate protein content
> Lower carbohydrate content than standard formulas
>
> Indications — May be effective in some enterally fed patients with difficult-to-control blood glucose
> Depending on level of kidney function and recommended use, micronutrient content should be evaluated closely
>
> ***Formulas specialized for chronic kidney disease***
>
> Example — Suplena[c] and Renalcal[b] (predialysis); Nepro[c] (on dialysis)
>
> Characteristics — 1.8 to 2 kcal/mL. Protein and electrolytes modified
>
> Indications — Useful in patients with difficult-to-control serum electrolyte levels

[a] Manufacturers may change product formulations and offerings. Check product labels and websites for the most current information.
[b] Manufactured by Nestlé Nutrition, Bridgewater Township, NJ 08807 (www.nestlehealthscience.us).
[c] Manufactured by Abbott Nutrition, Abbott Park, IL 60064 (http://abbottnutrition.com).

Nutrition Education

The *Abridged Nutrition Care Process Terminology (NCPT) Reference Manual*[1] and eNCPT[2] website define nutrition education as "a formal process to instruct or train a patient in a skill or to impart knowledge to help patients/clients voluntarily manage or modify food choices or eating behavior to maintain or improve health." Nutrition education is part of the nutrition intervention and has two subcategories[2]:

- nutrition education content
  - content-related nutrition education
  - education on nutrition's influence on health
  - physical activity guidance

- nutrition education application
  - nutrition-related laboratory result interpretation education
  - nutrition-related skill education
  - technical nutrition education

Suggested schedules for nutrition visits for medical nutrition therapy (MNT) in CKD have been published.[3-5] These schedules can be helpful in developing protocols for nutrition counseling and nutrition education. See Table 1.2 on page 5 for information about the number of annual MNT visits for CKD that are approved for reimbursement under Medicare Part B guidelines.

Box 5.3 on page 140 lists several major resources for nutrition education materials that target populations with CKD. The following brief discussions are intended to provide registered dietitian nutritionists (RDNs) with some suggested nutrition education topics and resources to support MNT recommendations from various evidence-based guidelines.

Weight Management

Weight Loss

Weight loss therapy, when appropriate, should be individualized. Discussions of label reading, alternative approaches to weight loss, and physical activity goals can be useful. For more information on physical activity, see Box 5.4 on page 142. Interventions to consider when patients with CKD need to lose weight include the following[6]:

- Increase activity as approved by the physician.
- Control energy intake to support weight loss.
- Reduce intake of sugars, fats, and foods of low nutrient density.
- Utilize food log and physical activity tracker applications such as MyFitnessPal or LoseIt.

BOX 5.3 Nutrition Education Resources for Chronic Kidney Disease[a]

Academy of Nutrition and Dietetics
Nutrition Care Manual

Comprehensive online clinical nutrition manual with professional information and patient handouts related to chronic kidney disease (CKD); subscription required.
www.nutritioncaremanual.org

Clinical Guide to Nutrition Care in Kidney Disease, 3rd edition
www.eatrightstore.org/product-type/ebooks/clinical-guide-to-nutrition-care-in-kidney-disease-3rd-edition

National Kidney Diet Professional Guide and Handouts, 3rd edition
www.eatrightstore.org/product-type/books/national-kidney-diet-professional-guide-handouts

National Kidney Diet: Dish Up a Kidney-Friendly Meal (patient education)
www.eatrightstore.org/product-type/booklets-and-handouts/national-kidney-diet-not-on-dialysis-dishup-a-kidneyfriendly-meal-for-patients-with-chronic-kidney-d

National Kidney Diet: Dish Up a Dialysis-Friendly Meal (patient education)
www.eatrightstore.org/product-type/booklets-and-handouts/national-kidney-diet-dishup-a-dialysisfriendly-meal-for-patients-with-chronic-kidney-disease-on-dial

American Association of Kidney Patients
A nonprofit company; "The independent voice of kidney patients since 1969." *aakpRENALIFE* magazine is available free online; membership is free for patients and family members
www.aakp.org/join

Journal of Renal Nutrition, *Collections, Patient Education Papers*
Professional publication of the National Kidney Foundation—Council on Renal Nutrition; member log-in not required
www.jrnjournal.org/content/patienteducation

MedLine Plus
From the US National Library of Medicine and the US National Institutes of Health
www.nlm.nih.gov/medlineplus/kidneyfailure.html

> **BOX 5.3   Nutrition Education Resources for Chronic Kidney Disease (cont.)[a]**
>
> ### Life Options
> A program of the Medical Education Institute; includes links for Kidney School (interactive modules for patients with CKD) and Home Dialysis Central (information about home dialysis in all modalities)
> www.lifeoptions.org
>
> ### National Kidney Disease Education Program
> Home page from the US Department of Health and Human Services and the National Institute of Diabetes and Digestive and Kidney Diseases.
> www.nkdep.nih.gov/professionals/index.htm
>
> Nutrition materials for professionals and patients
> www.nkdep.nih.gov/professionals/ckd-nutrition.htm
>
> ### National Kidney Foundation
> Home page
> www.kidney.org
>
> *Pocket Guide to Nutrition Assessment of the Patient with Kidney Disease*, 6th edition
> www.kidney.org/professionals/CRN/ClinicalTools
>
> Nutrition and diet information for patients
> www.kidney.org/nutrition
>
> ### Renal Dietitians Dietetic Practice Group of the Academy of Nutrition and Dietetics
> Patient education materials available to group members only
> www.renalnutrition.org
>
> ### Websites of dialysis providers
> Many materials are proprietary and subject to change; dietitians encouraged to check for materials as needed.

[a] This list is not meant to be all-inclusive. It identifies major sources of materials that are useful in nutrition education and counseling related to chronic kidney disease or end-stage renal disease.

BOX 5.4 Physical Activity Guidelines

Adults

Adults should move more and sit less. Some physical activity is better than none. Adults who sit less and do any amount of moderate-to-vigorous physical activity gain some health benefits.

For substantial health benefits, adults should do at least 150 to 300 minutes a week of moderate-intensity[a] or 75 to 150 minutes a week of vigorous-intensity[b] aerobic physical activity. Aerobic exercise should preferably be spread throughout the week.

Additional health benefits are gained by engaging in physical activity beyond the equivalent of 300 minutes of moderate-intensity physical activity a week.

Incorporate muscle-strengthening activity[c] of moderate or greater intensity and that involves all major muscle groups 2 or more days a week.

Older adults

The guidelines for adults also apply to older adults.

Older adults should incorporate balance training in addition to aerobic and muscle-strengthening activities.

Older adults with chronic conditions should understand whether and how their conditions affect their ability to do regular physical activity safely.

If older adults cannot complete 150 minutes of physical activity a week because of chronic conditions, they should be as physically active as their abilities and conditions allow.

Pregnant adults

Complete at least 150 minutes of moderate-intensity aerobic activity a week during pregnancy and the postpartum period. Aerobic activity should preferably be spread throughout the week.

Individuals who habitually engaged in vigorous-intensity aerobic activity or who were physically active before pregnancy can continue these activities during pregnancy and the postpartum period.

Individuals who are pregnant can consult with their health care provider about whether or how to adjust their physical activity during pregnancy and the postpartum period.

> **BOX 5.4 Physical Activity Guidelines (cont.)**
>
> ***Adults with chronic conditions and disabilities***
>
> As able, adults with chronic conditions or disabilities should do at least 150 to 300 minutes a week of moderate-intensity or 75 to 150 minutes a week of vigorous-intensity aerobic physical activity. Aerobic exercise should preferably be spread throughout the week.
>
> As able, adults with chronic conditions or disabilities should incorporate muscle-strengthening activity of moderate or greater intensity and that involve all major muscle groups 2 or more days a week.
>
> When adults with chronic conditions or disabilities are not able to meet the above guidelines, they should engage in regular physical activity according to their abilities and should avoid inactivity.
>
> Individuals with chronic conditions can consult a health care professional or physical activity specialist about the types and amounts of activity appropriate for their abilities and conditions.

Adapted from US Department of Health and Human Services. *Physical Activity Guidelines for Americans.* 2nd ed. US Department of Health and Human Services; 2018. Accessed September 6, 2023. https://health.gov/paguidelines/second-edition/pdf/Physical_Activity_Guidelines_2nd_edition.pdf

[a] Moderate-intensity activity examples include walking briskly or doubles tennis.
[b] Vigorous-intensity activity examples include jogging, running, shoveling snow, or a strenuous fitness class.
[c] Muscle-strengthening activity examples include resistance training, weight lifting, or calisthenics.

- Refer to formal weight management program and/or physical therapy when appropriate.
- If the patient is on peritoneal dialysis (PD), also consider:
  - limiting sodium and fluid to reduce the need for higher-percentage dextrose exchanges, or
  - alternate osmotic agents, such as icodextrin.

Weight Gain

If patients are underweight, RDNs can work with them to identify means to improve energy intake. Appetite stimulants may also be appropriate, although it is important to understand their potential adverse effects (see Box 5.5 on page 144).

> **BOX 5.5 Appetite Stimulants and Their Adverse Effects**
>
> **Megestrol acetate (Megace[a])**
> Constipation, diarrhea, dyspepsia, hyperglycemia, nausea, and vomiting
> Blood clots in sedentary individuals
>
> **Dronabinol (Marinol[b])**
> Seizure and seizure-like activity
> Abdominal pain, dizziness, euphoria, somnolence, paranoia, tachycardia, and central nervous system effects (amnesia, changes in mood, confusion, delusions, hallucinations, mental depression, nervousness, or anxiety)
> Sleep disturbances may occur after discontinuation of therapy
>
> **Mirtazapine (Remeron[c])**
> Abnormal dreams and/or thinking, dizziness, drowsiness, constipation, flu-like symptoms, dry mouth, increased appetite, and weight gain
>
> **Note:** This drug is an antidepressant that may be used for appetite stimulation because of its side effects of increased appetite and weight gain.

Adapted with permission from de Waal D. Medications commonly prescribed in kidney disease. In: Phillips S, Gonyea J, eds. *Clinical Guide to Nutrition Care in Kidney Disease*. 3rd ed. Academy of Nutrition and Dietetics; 2022:371.
[a] Manufactured by Par Pharmaceutical Companies Inc, Spring Valley, NY.
[b] Manufactured by Sovay Pharmaceuticals Neder-Over-Heembeek, Brussels, Belgium.
[c] Manufactured by Organon USA Inc, Jersey City, NJ.

Protein, Fat, Carbohydrate, and Fiber Intake

Exchange lists that include macronutrients and micronutrients of concern in renal nutrition can be useful in patient education (see Table 5.1).

Box 4.5 on page 93 summarizes MNT priorities for patients on hemodialysis (HD) and PD, including goals for dietary fat. Education materials from the National Heart, Lung, and Blood Institute (www.nhlbi.nih.gov/resources/about) can be applied in CKD, with modification as needed for the special needs of this population.

Carbohydrate intake may be addressed as part of nutrition education for patients with CKD and diabetes. Box 5.6 on page 146 presents guidelines for integrating CKD and diabetes education.[7]

TABLE 5.1 National Renal Diet Exchanges for Chronic Kidney Disease[a]

Food group	Protein, g	Energy, kcal	Na, mg	K, mg	PO$_4$, mg
Protein	6-8	50-100	20-150	50-150	50-100
High PO$_4$ protein	6-8	50-100	20-150	50-350	100-300
High Na protein	6-8	50-100	200-450	50-150	50-100
Vegetarian protein	6-8	70-150	10-200	60-150	80-150
High Na/K/PO$_4$	6-8	70-150	250-400	250-500	200-400
Vegetables					
Low K	2-3	10-100	0-50	20-150	10-70
Medium K	2-3	10-100	0-50	150-250	10-70
High K	2-3	10-100	0-50	250-550	10-70
Fruit					
Low K	0-1	20-100	0-10	20-150	1-20
Medium K	0-1	20-100	0-10	150-250	1-20
High K	0-1	20-100	0-10	250-550	1-20
Breads and starches	2-3	50-200	0-150	10-100	10-70
High Na, PO$_4$	2-3	50-200	150-400	10-100	100-200
Calorie boosters	0-1	100-150	0-100	0-100	0-100
Flavor	0	0-20	250-300	0-100	0-20

Abbreviations: Na, sodium; K, potassium, PO$_4$, phosphorus
Adapted with permission from American Dietetic Association. *National Renal Diet: Professional Guide.* 2nd ed. American Dietetic Association; 2002.
[a] Nutrient information is per serving.

As a result of restrictions on dietary phosphorus intake, many patients with CKD have difficulty achieving adequate intake of dietary fiber. Natural foods contain organic phosphorus, whereas inorganic phosphorus is the form used as an additive in foods. Organic

> **BOX 5.6 Components and Principles of Diabetes and Chronic Kidney Disease Self-Management**
>
> Describe the disease processes for diabetes and chronic kidney disease (CKD) as well as treatment options.
>
> Provide explanations in lay terminology and evaluate the patient's understanding. Assess and address beliefs about the nature, cause, and treatment of the illness. Explain risks and consequences of nonadherence.
>
> Promote social support by involving significant others in educational activities.
>
> Incorporate appropriate nutritional management. Attention should be paid to cultural food preferences in nutrition counseling.
>
> Describe purpose and side effects of medicines. Include caregivers. Explain that health care providers and the patient work together to find the right treatment regimen.
>
> Discuss importance of self-monitoring of glucose. Describe symptoms of hyper- and hypoglycemia. Assess patient awareness of hypoglycemia.
>
> Review prevention, detection, and treatment of further diabetes complications.
>
> Encourage risk reduction behavior such as smoking cessation, exercise, weight loss, and continued management of nutrition and medications.
>
> Support problem solving and goal setting. Establish a stepwise approach to easily achievable goals. Encourage discussion of barriers (eg, transportation, financial issues, social support) and refer as appropriate.
>
> Integrate psychosocial evaluation and refer as appropriate.
>
> Promote preconception care, management during pregnancy, and gestational diabetes management as appropriate.

Adapted with permission from Kidney Disease Outcomes Quality Initiative. KDOQI clinical practice guidelines and clinical practice recommendations for diabetes and chronic kidney disease. *Am J Kidney Dis.* 2007;49(2 suppl 2):S12-S154.

phosphorus is absorbed at 40% to 60% from animal sources and at 20% to 50% from plant-based foods. Inorganic phosphate additives can be absorbed up to 100%.[8] Helpful nutrition education tools are available on the websites of some dialysis providers or on other internet sites as noted in Box 5.3.

Sodium, Potassium, Phosphorus, and Other Minerals

Recommendations for sodium, potassium, phosphorus, and other minerals for different stages of the CKD spectrum and for different modalities of renal replacement therapy are summarized in Chapter 4. Exchange lists for renal diets can be used to teach patients how to select foods when sodium, potassium, and phosphorus must be controlled (see Table 5.1). RDNs can make further adjustments to address individual economic, cultural, and other considerations.

Phosphorus

Nutrition education for phosphorus control in CKD stage 5 can inform patients about food sources of phosphorus and enable them to adjust phosphorus-binder doses according to intake (see Box 2.2 on page 19 for basic information about binders). Foods with natural phosphorus should be encouraged over those with added phosphorus, since the total amount absorbed is less.

Calcium

RDNs can provide practical advice to patients with CKD about how to achieve recommended goals for calcium intake of less than 2,000 mg/d.[3] The RDN should educate patients about calcium from all sources, including diet and medications such as phosphorus binders (see Box 2.2).

Iron

Patients may be instructed to take iron supplements to maintain adequate serum iron levels. See Table 5.2 on page 148 for more information on common iron supplements.[9]

Vitamins

The evidenced-based nutrition practice guidelines for CKD provide detailed recommendations for vitamin B intake as well as vitamin C.

TABLE 5.2 Common Oral Iron Supplements

Selected product (Iron compound)	Percentage of elemental iron
Ferrous fumarate (Ferro-Sequels,[a] Hemocyte, Nephro-Fer)	33
Ferrous gluconate (FE-40, Fergon)	12
Ferrous sulfate (Feosol, tablet or capsule; Slow Fe)	20
Heme iron polypeptide (Proferrin)	Not available (12 mg elemental iron per tablet)
Iron polysaccharide complex (EzFe, Ferrex 150, Niferex, Niferex-150)	100

[a] Contains docusate.
Adapted with permission from McCann L. *Pocket Guide to Nutrition Assessment of the Patient with Kidney Disease*. 6th ed. National Kidney Foundation; 2021.

See the Appendix on page 184 for information about some common preparations of renal-specific multivitamins. The RDN can inform patients about standards to assess vitamin D nutrition in CKD and about recommended repletion of vitamin D in accordance with the practice guidelines for CKD.[3] See Chapter 4 for additional information on vitamins and CKD.

Medications and Food Safety After Kidney Transplant

Immunosuppressants for individuals who have had a kidney transplant have numerous adverse effects that may respond to nutrition interventions (see Box 5.7).[4] Patients who have received a transplant are at increased risk of foodborne illness and should be carefully educated about basic food safety (see Box 5.8 on page 151).[10]

BOX 5.7 Potential Nutrition-Related Adverse Effects of Immunosuppressants and Possible Interventions

Cyclosporin A (Sandimmune, Neoral[a])

Hyperkalemia	Restrict potassium intake
Hyperglycemia	Monitor blood glucose levels; address carbohydrate load and distribution
Gingival hyperplasia	Encourage good oral hygiene
Hypertension	Restrict sodium intake
Hypomagnesemia	Suggest magnesium supplements
Gastrointestinal distress	Provide nutrient-dense foods that patient will eat; ensure adequate protein and fluid intake
Hyperlipidemia	Suggest therapeutic lifestyle changes

Azathioprine (Imuran[b])

Infection	Provide nutrient-dense foods that patient will eat
Mouth ulcers	Modify diet texture
Folate deficiency	Suggest folate supplements
Gastrointestinal distress	Provide nutrient-dense foods that patient will eat; ensure adequate protein and fluid intake

Corticosteroids (Prednisone[c], Prednisolone[c], Solu-Medrol[d])

Cushingoid appearance	Address carbohydrate load and increase protein intake
Sodium retention	Restrict sodium intake
Enhanced appetite	Suggest low-calorie snacks and eating behavior modification

Continued on next page

BOX 5.7 Potential Nutrition-Related Adverse Effects of Immunosuppressants and Possible Interventions (cont.)

Corticosteroids (Prednisone[c], Prednisolone[c], Solu-Medrol[d]) (continued)

Hyperlipidemia	Limit fat intake to less than 30% calories during long-term phase
Hyperglycemia	Monitor blood glucose levels; address carbohydrate load and distribution
Protein catabolism	Increase protein provision
Gastrointestinal ulceration	Limit/restrict caffeine if patient has caffeine sensitivity
Bone loss	Ensure adequate calcium and vitamin D intake; consider need for bisphosphonates, calcitriol, and estrogen or testosterone

Tacrolimus (Prograf, FK506[e])

Hypertension	Restrict sodium intake
Hyperglycemia	Monitor blood glucose levels and address carbohydrate load and distribution
Hyperlipidemia	Limit fat intake to less than 30% calories during long-term phase
Hyperkalemia	Restrict potassium intake
Hypomagnesemia	Suggest magnesium supplements
Gastrointestinal distress	Provide nutrient-dense foods that patient will eat; ensure adequate protein and fluid intake

Mycophenolate mofetil (Cellcept, RS-61443[f]), antithymocyte globulin (ATG[g]), muromonab-CD3 (Orthoclone OKT3[h]), daclizumab (Zenapax[f]), and basiliximab (Simulect[a])

Gastrointestinal distress	Provide nutrient-dense foods that patient will eat; ensure adequate protein and fluid intake

BOX 5.7 Potential Nutrition-Related Adverse Effects of Immunosuppressants and Possible Interventions (cont.)

Sirolimus (Rapamune[j])

Hyperlipidemia	Monitor blood glucose levels; address carbohydrate load and distribution
Delayed wound healing	Suggest vitamin supplementation and increased protein intake
Hypokalemia	Suggest potassium supplements

Manufacturers are as follows: [a] Novartis Pharmaceuticals, East Hanover, NJ 07936; [b] Bedford Laboratories, Bedford, OH 44146; [c] Rixabe Laboratories, Columbus, OH 43228; [d] Pfizer, New York, NY 10017; [e] Astellas Pharma US, Deerfield, IL 60015; [f] Novartis Pharmaceuticals, East Hanover, NJ; [g] Upjohn, Kalamazoo, MI 49001; [h] Ortho Biotech, Bridgewater, NJ 08807-0914; [i] Wyeth Pharmaceuticals, Philadelphia, PA 19101.

Adapted with permission from Norris H, Cochran C. Nutrition management of the adult kidney transplant patient. In: Phillips S, Gonyea J, eds. *Clinical Guide to Nutrition Care in Kidney Disease*. 3rd ed. Academy of Nutrition and Dietetics; 2022:115-116.

BOX 5.8 Food Safety Recommendations for Immunosuppressed Individuals

Avoid the following:

- All raw and undercooked meats (especially ground or chopped), poultry, fish, and game
- Sushi, raw seafood, and shellfish
- Raw or undercooked eggs and foods containing them (eg, homemade eggnog, Caesar dressing)
- All unpasteurized milk and dairy products
- Unpasteurized juices and ciders
- All fresh, uncooked sprouts (bean, alfalfa, others)
- Raw or spoiled food items
- Food contaminated with a foodborne illness
- Outdated packaged foods
- Food from dented or otherwise damaged containers

Continued on next page

> **BOX 5.8 Food Safety Recommendations for Immunosuppressed Individuals (cont.)**
>
> Always practice the following:
> - Use safe food-handling methods (see www.foodsafety.gov).
> - Store food promptly and appropriately.
> - Use leftovers within 1 to 2 days.
> - Avoid buffet-style meals, salad bars, and potlucks.
> - Drink water from safe sources.

Adapted from US Department of Agriculture. *Food Safety: A Need-to-Know Guide for Those at Risk*. Revised 2020. www.fsis.usda.gov/sites/default/files/media_file/2021-04/at-risk-booklet.pdf

Nutrition Counseling

In the nutrition counseling domain, the RDN's intervention moves beyond strengthening the patient's knowledge base to helping the patient set priorities and develop behaviors that support ongoing care. In the *NCPT Reference Manual: Standardized Terminology for the Nutrition Care Process*, nutrition counseling is described as "a supportive process, characterized by a collaborative counselor-patient relationship to establish food, nutrition and physical activity priorities, goals, and individualized action plans that acknowledge and foster responsibility for self-care to treat an existing condition and promote health."[1]

The material in this section has been adapted from the second edition of the *Academy of Nutrition and Dietetics Pocket Guide to Lipid Disorders, Hypertension, Diabetes, and Weight Management*[11] and summarizes an organized approach to evaluate patient readiness for counseling and to determine appropriate behavior-change strategies.

The *5 A's* describe steps that can guide the RDN in starting an education/counseling session and implementing the best of several behavioral change strategies for each part of the session[12]:

- Step 1: Ask
- Step 2: Assess
- Step 3: Advise

- Step 4: Agree
- Step 5: Arrange

Taken together, these 5 A's provide a workable framework that can integrate other counseling models.

Step 1: Ask

The *ask* step emphasizes the importance of asking questions as the RDN aims to develop a relationship with the patient. The following tactics are essential to this step[11]:

- Use motivational interviewing techniques (see Box 5.9) throughout the nutrition education/counseling session.[11,13,14]
- Establish rapport by demonstrating the ability to be open, genuine, caring, and empathetic.
- Begin each session by asking questions to determine what the patient wants to know and accomplish and what you can do to be of assistance.

BOX 5.9 Motivational Interviewing Techniques[11,13,14]

Ask open-ended questions
Encourage patients to do the talking.
Do not ask questions that elicit a "yes" or "no" response.

Express empathy
Acknowledge the patient's difficulties.
Validate the patient's thoughts and feelings.

Listen reflectively
Rephrase the patient's responses to reflect what you think you heard.
State back what you think the patient meant.

Support self-efficacy
Provide choices and reassure the patient about expected outcomes.

Continued on next page

> **BOX 5.9   Motivational Interviewing Techniques (cont.)[11,13,14]**
>
> **Express sympathy**
> Express acceptance and understanding.
> Use reflective listening and expect ambivalence.
>
> **Explore discrepancies**
> Let individuals explore their reasons for changing or not changing behaviors.
>
> **Roll with resistance**
> Avoid arguments.
> Avoid judging and labeling.
> Change strategies if individuals show resistance.
>
> **Summarize**
> Rephrase the overall content and meaning of the conversation.
> Reveal any ambiguity.
>
> **Promote empowerment**
> Recognize that individuals are the source of their own solutions, and each individual is in charge of and responsible for their own care.

Step 2: Assess

In the *assess* step, the RDN evaluates the patient's readiness to change (see Box 5.10)[11,15] as part of the nutrition assessment (see Chapter 2 for more information on nutrition assessment).

When using the stages of change, the RDN's objective is to help the patient achieve the action or maintenance stage for the desired behavior[11]:

- If patients are in the **precontemplation** stage, the goal is to help them recognize that they are at risk for a health problem.
- If patients are in the **contemplation** stage, aim to help them believe their risk of disease is serious and that personal actions make a difference. The benefits must outweigh the barriers to patients before they will take the next step.

- If patients are in the **preparation** stage, provide encouragement and set a start date.
- If patients are in the **action** stage, help them implement the strategies that individuals who have made lifestyle changes identify as the most helpful (see Box 5.11 on page 157).[11,16] Use tools such as:
  - food and activity records so the patient becomes aware of changes they need and are willing to make (also helpful in the preparation stage), or
  - goal setting so the patient determines to make realistic changes.
- If patients are in the **maintenance** stage, provide support and continue encouragement to facilitate behaviors that maintain the healthful change (see Box 5.12 on page 158).[11,17]

BOX 5.10 Transtheoretical Model of Intentional Behavior Change (Stages of Change)[11,17]

Precontemplation

Attitude toward lifestyle change: Never

Patient has no intention of changing behavior in foreseeable future. They are unaware of problem or resistant to efforts to modify behavior.

Interventions for health professionals:
- Personalize risk factors.
- Discuss health concern(s) and implications.

Contemplation

Attitude toward lifestyle change: Someday

Patient is aware there is a problem and is seriously thinking about change, but has no commitment to action in near future.

Interventions for health professionals:
- Provide basic information.
- Demonstrate that the pros of change outweigh the cons.

Continued on next page

BOX 5.10 Transtheoretical Model of Intentional Behavior Change (Stages of Change) (cont.)[11,17]

Preparation

Attitude toward lifestyle change: Soon

Patient is prepared to make decisions and is committed to action in the next 30 days; they begin small behavioral changes.

Interventions for health professionals:
- Establish a start date.
- Teach specific "how-to" skills.

Action

Attitude toward lifestyle change: Now

Patient demonstrates notable overt efforts to change and targets behaviors that can be modified to acceptable criteria. They may not consistently carry out new behaviors.

Interventions for health professionals:
- Implement counseling strategies.
- Continue to reinforce and support decision to change.
- Discuss difference between a lapse and a relapse.

Maintenance

Attitude toward lifestyle change: Forever

Patient is working to stabilize behavior change and avoid relapse and maintains behavior change for at least 6 months.

Interventions for health professionals:
- Provide support; encourage behavior maintenance strategies.
- Continue relapse prevention counseling.

BOX 5.11 Strategies for Modifying Behavior[11,16]

Self-monitoring
Record target behaviors and associated factors to increase awareness of behavior; participants report this strategy to be helpful.

Record the "what, where, and when" of eating and physical activity (individuals with diabetes should also keep blood glucose monitoring records).

Goal setting
Set specific short-term targets for behavior habits to achieve incremental improvements.

Stimulus control
Identify triggers for problem behaviors; design strategies to break links.

Restrict environmental factors associated with inappropriate behaviors.

Eat at specific times; set aside time and place for physical activities.

Avoid purchasing foods that are perceived as difficult to eat in moderation.

Cognitive restructuring
Change perceptions, thoughts, or beliefs that undermine behavior-change efforts.

Change thinking patterns from unrealistic goals to realistic and achievable goals.

Move thinking patterns away from self-rejection and toward self-acceptance.

Contingency management
Use rewards (tangible or verbal) to improve performance of specific behaviors or recognize when specified goals are reached (participants rated this strategy as least helpful).

Create contracts to formalize agreements; contracts should be short term and focus on increasing healthful behaviors.

Stress management
Stress is a primary predictor of relapse; therefore, methods to reduce stress and tension are critical.

Try tension reduction skills such as diaphragmatic breathing, progressive muscle relaxation, and/or meditation.

Regular physical activity helps reduce stress.

> **BOX 5.12 Strategies for Maintaining Behavior Change[11,17]**
>
> **Structured programs with ongoing contact**
> Individuals aiming to achieve and maintain goals require assistance from structured programs with consistent follow-up contacts.
>
> Maintain visits, telephone calls, or internet communication to promote adherence with recommended lifestyle changes.
>
> **Social support**
> Use social support—family, peer support, self-help or worksite groups, or involvement in social activities—to maintain successful behavior change.
>
> **Physical activity and exercise**
> Promote regular involvement in physical activities—individuals who exercise regularly are also more likely to maintain other health behaviors.
>
> **Relapse prevention**
> Recognize that lapses in behavior can be anticipated in certain situations (eg, travel, social situations, celebrations, stressful situations, loneliness) and develop skills for those situations.
>
> Individuals can practice coping strategies to handle high-risk situations (eg, stress management, social situation skills).

Step 3: Advise

The *advise* step uses a patient-centered framework as follows[11]:

- Focus on the concerns of the patient.
- Allow the patient to be the expert for themselves.
- Adapt nutrition interventions to meet the patient's needs, wants, priorities, preferences, and expectations.

Step 4: Agree

In the *agree* step, the RDN facilitates the patient's process of setting their own short-term goals related to nutrition, physical activity, or monitoring of pertinent laboratory tests (as appropriate) and helps outline the patient's potential methods for accomplishing a lifestyle change. Scaling questions are recommended. Following are some examples[11]:

- To evaluate a patient's goals: "On a scale of 0 to 10, with 0 being not important and 10 being very important, how important is it for you to modify XX behavior?"
- To evaluate a patient's plans: "On a scale of 0 to 10, with 0 being not confident and 10 being very confident, how confident are you that you can XX?"

Step 5: Arrange

In the *arrange* step, the RDN helps implement a plan for follow-up adapted to the patient's goals and needs, the patient's level of support from family and friends, and the available resources.[6] Crucial tasks include the following[6]:

- Schedule follow-up visits.
- Provide contact information for future questions.
- Make referrals and/or provide contact information for other providers.

Coordination of Nutrition Care

The fourth domain of nutrition intervention is defined as "consultation with, referral to, or coordination of nutrition care with other health care providers, institutions, or agencies that can assist in treating or managing nutrition-related problems."[1] Given the long-term relationship between RDNs in dialysis centers and their patients, there can be many intervention opportunities over the years in this domain. Professional partners in coordinated care may include staff at home health agencies and long-term-care facilities, health care professionals specializing in diabetes care, RDNs working in community settings such as Meals on Wheels, or RDNs in other specialties such as weight management, liver disease, and other areas.

Case Study

Nutrition Care Process

Step 3: Nutrition Intervention

Part 2: Implementation

> This chapter adds the second part of the nutrition intervention piece of the NCP to information captured in the assessment presented in Chapter 2, development of the diagnosis presented in Chapter 3, and planning of the nutrition prescription presented in Chapter 4. New information is set off from the previous material in white. This chapter addresses the nutrition intervention domains of nutrition education and nutrition counseling. Although coordination of care is not an intervention at this time, it may be addressed in future documentation.

A 56-year-old female individual with CKD stage 5D on peritoneal dialysis is admitted to the hospital.

Nutrition Assessment

Food/Nutrition-Related History

Food Intake
Patient consumes traditional Cambodian foods and follows traditional Cambodian meal patterns, including rice, stir-fried vegetables, and

small amounts of fish, poultry, and beef. Uses fish sauce frequently. Has been consuming increased amounts of cola soft drinks to ease nausea.

Medications
HMG-CoA reductase inhibitor (statin), renal multivitamin, calcium carbonate and sevelamer with meals, calcitriol, ferrous sulfate, insulin aspart with meals, isoniazid, vitamin B6, and lansoprazole. Has missed a few days of taking medications because of current condition.

Food and Nutrition Knowledge/Skill
Family is aware of low phosphorus and low potassium foods; is very involved.

Physical activity
Sedentary

Anthropometric Measurements

Body Composition, Growth, and Weight History

Height
150 cm (59 in)

Admit weight
74.5 kg (164 lb)

Estimated dry weight (EDW)
72 kg (has been stable)

BMI (using EDW)
32

Frame size
Medium

Ideal body weight (IBW)
62 kg; 116% IBW

Biochemical Data, Medical Tests, and Procedures

Electrolyte and renal profile
See laboratory data table.

Nutritional anemia profile
See laboratory data table.

Urine output
500 mL/24 h

Laboratory Data for Nutrition Assessment of Patient[3]

Laboratory test	Reference range	Patient result
Potassium, mmol/L	Normal: 3.4-5 Peritoneal dialysis (PD)[a]: 3.5-5.5	5.4
Blood urea nitrogen, mg/dL	Normal: 6-20 PD: >60	58
Creatinine, mg/dL	Normal: 0.7-1.3 PD: not defined	11
Glucose, mg/dL	Normal (fasting): 60-99	92
Calcium, mg/dL	Normal: 8.6-10.2	8.8
Phosphorus, mg/dL	Normal: 2.4-4.7 PD: 3.5-5.5	5.7
Albumin, g/dL	Normal: 3.5-4.7 PD: >3.5	1.6
Hemoglobin, g/dL	Normal: 13.5-17.5 PD: 10-12	9
Capillary blood glucose, mg/dL	Normal: <150	120-250
Sodium, mmol/L	Normal: 134-143	129

[a] Reference range for patients on peritoneal dialysis.

Nutrition Focused Physical Findings

- Overall appearance: abrasions on arms and neck from scratching
- Obese with central adiposity
- Bilateral ankle edema and edema of eyelid
- Diarrhea, nausea, and vomiting
- Pale conjunctiva
- Koilonychia (spoon-shaped nails)

Patient History

Personal data: Patient is 56-year-old female individual, does not speak English; children are fluent in English and are very involved and supportive.

Patient or family nutrition-oriented medical/health history: ESRD due to hypertension. History includes type 2 diabetes. Admitted to the hospital with peritonitis, pain, nausea, vomiting, and fever. Third episode of peritonitis in 2 months. Latent tuberculosis.

Treatment/therapy: Peritoneal dialysis with five exchanges per day, each 2 L 2.5% dextrose. Type 2 diabetes mellitus managed with insulin; capillary blood glucose usually less than 250 mg/dL.

Nutrition Diagnosis

Intake Domain

Nutrition Diagnosis
Excessive mineral intake (sodium)

Sample PES Statement
Excessive sodium intake related to cultural food patterns as evidenced by diet recall revealing frequent use of fish sauce as well as presence of ankle and orbital edema.

Clinical Domain

Nutrition Diagnosis

Altered nutrition-related laboratory values (serum phosphorus and albumin)

Sample PES Statements

- Altered nutrition-related laboratory values (serum phosphorus) related to missed binder doses as evidenced by patient report and serum phosphorus value of 5.7 mg/dL.
- Altered nutrition-related laboratory values (serum albumin) related to altered nutrient utilization in inflammatory state as evidenced by serum albumin of 1.6 g/dL in a patient with acute peritonitis.

Behavioral-Environmental Domain

Nutrition Diagnosis

Limited adherence to nutrition-related recommendations.

Sample PES Statement

Limited adherence to nutrition-related recommendations related to the use of high-phosphorus soft drinks to treat gastrointestinal symptoms as evidenced by patient reports of drinking cola beverages during episodes of nausea.

Nutrition Intervention

Peritoneal Dialysis Regimen

Patient receives PD with five exchanges per day, each 2 L 2.5% dextrose.

Note: 2.5% dextrose provides 25 g dextrose/L (see Table 4.7 on page 111 for additional information on dextrose contributions).

Calculate calories from daily PD exchanges as follows:

$$2 \text{ L per exchange} \times (25 \text{ g dextrose/L}) = 50 \text{ g dextrose per PD exchange}$$

$$(50 \text{ g dextrose per PD exchange}) \times (5 \text{ PD exchanges/d}) = 250 \text{ g dextrose/d}$$

$$(250 \text{ g dextrose/d}) \times (3.4 \text{ kcal/g dextrose}) = 850 \text{ kcal/d}$$

$$(850 \text{ kcal/d}) \times 70\% \text{ absorption} = 595 \text{ kcal/d from PD exchanges}$$

Calculating Energy and Protein Needs

Note: Calculation uses dry weight
Energy needs:

$$72 \text{ kg} \times 25 \text{ to } 30 \text{ kcal/kg/d} = 1,800 \text{ to } 2,160 \text{ kcal/d}$$

Subtract 595 kcal provided by PD regimen = 1,205 to 1,565 kcal/d

Protein needs (increased due to peritonitis):

$$72 \text{ kg} \times 1.3 \text{ g/kg/d} = 94 \text{ g/d}$$

Daily Nutrition Prescription for Patient Undergoing Peritoneal Dialysis

Other elements of the nutrition prescription are as follows:

- Based on the patient's past medical history and calculated macronutrient and micronutrient needs, suggest a renal, carbohydrate-controlled diet adjusted to cultural food preferences as permissible within renal and diabetic requirements.
- Based on urine output of 500 mL/24 h and edema/hyponatremia, suggest limiting dietary fluid intake to 1,000 mL/d.
- Based on edema/hyponatremia, suggest limiting dietary sodium to approximately 2.3 g/d.

- Based on hyperphosphatemia, adjust dietary phosphorus intake, including phosphorus additives, to reduce phosphorus within normal range. Confirm patient is taking phosphorus binders with meals.
- To prevent undesirable weight gain while maintaining dry weight, limit dietary calories to approximately 1,600 kcal/d. (Patient will receive an additional 595 kcal/d from PD exchanges.)
- To replete protein stores in the context of peritonitis, provide approximately 94 g protein per day. Reevaluate adequacy of estimated protein needs at nutrition follow-up.

Nutrition Intervention: Education

Explain to the patient the nutrition modifications needed to reduce fluid and sodium intake due to the presence of edema and hyponatremia.

Explain to the patient the nutrition modifications needed to reduce dietary phosphorus. Help the patient identify different methods to control nausea symptoms, such as switching to a carbonated beverage that is *not* cola to reduce phosphorus intake and eating a moderate amount of low-sodium crackers.

Explain to the patient that she is absorbing additional calories from the peritoneal dialysate and that intake of oral calories will need to be adjusted accordingly to prevent excessive weight gain.

Explain to the patient that her protein needs have increased because of peritonitis, while also educating her about the need to keep her phosphorus intake as low as possible.

Explain findings from laboratory tests and teach the patient how she can adjust her diet in accordance with laboratory results.

Nutrition Focused Physical Findings

- Overall appearance: abrasions on arms and neck from scratching
- Obese with central adiposity
- Bilateral ankle edema and edema of eyelid
- Diarrhea, nausea, and vomiting
- Pale conjunctiva
- Koilonychia (spoon-shaped nails)

Patient History

Personal data: Patient is 56-year-old female individual, does not speak English; children are fluent in English and are very involved and supportive.

Patient or family nutrition-oriented medical/health history: ESRD due to hypertension. History includes type 2 diabetes. Admitted to the hospital with peritonitis, pain, nausea, vomiting, and fever. Third episode of peritonitis in 2 months. Latent tuberculosis.

Treatment/therapy: Peritoneal dialysis with five exchanges per day, each 2 L 2.5% dextrose. Type 2 diabetes mellitus managed with insulin; capillary blood glucose usually less than 250 mg/dL.

Nutrition Diagnosis

Intake Domain

Nutrition Diagnosis
Excessive mineral intake (sodium)

Sample PES Statement
Excessive sodium intake related to cultural food patterns as evidenced by diet recall revealing frequent use of fish sauce as well as presence of ankle and orbital edema.

Clinical Domain

Nutrition Diagnosis

Altered nutrition-related laboratory values (serum phosphorus and albumin)

Sample PES Statements

- Altered nutrition-related laboratory values (serum phosphorus) related to missed binder doses as evidenced by patient report and serum phosphorus value of 5.7 mg/dL.
- Altered nutrition-related laboratory values (serum albumin) related to altered nutrient utilization in inflammatory state as evidenced by serum albumin of 1.6 g/dL in a patient with acute peritonitis.

Behavioral-Environmental Domain

Nutrition Diagnosis

Limited adherence to nutrition-related recommendations.

Sample PES Statement

Limited adherence to nutrition-related recommendations related to the use of high-phosphorus soft drinks to treat gastrointestinal symptoms as evidenced by patient reports of drinking cola beverages during episodes of nausea.

Nutrition Intervention

Peritoneal Dialysis Regimen

Patient receives PD with five exchanges per day, each 2 L 2.5% dextrose.

Note: 2.5% dextrose provides 25 g dextrose/L (see Table 4.7 on page 111 for additional information on dextrose contributions).

Calculate calories from daily PD exchanges as follows:

2 L per exchange × (25 g dextrose/L) = 50 g dextrose per PD exchange

(50 g dextrose per PD exchange) × (5 PD exchanges/d) = 250 g dextrose/d

(250 g dextrose/d) × (3.4 kcal/g dextrose) = 850 kcal/d

(850 kcal/d) × 70% absorption = 595 kcal/d from PD exchanges

Calculating Energy and Protein Needs

Note: Calculation uses dry weight
Energy needs:

72 kg × 25 to 30 kcal/kg/d = 1,800 to 2,160 kcal/d

Subtract 595 kcal provided by PD regimen = 1,205 to 1,565 kcal/d

Protein needs (increased due to peritonitis):

72 kg × 1.3 g/kg/d = 94 g/d

Daily Nutrition Prescription for Patient Undergoing Peritoneal Dialysis

Other elements of the nutrition prescription are as follows:

- Based on the patient's past medical history and calculated macronutrient and micronutrient needs, suggest a renal, carbohydrate-controlled diet adjusted to cultural food preferences as permissible within renal and diabetic requirements.
- Based on urine output of 500 mL/24 h and edema/hyponatremia, suggest limiting dietary fluid intake to 1,000 mL/d.
- Based on edema/hyponatremia, suggest limiting dietary sodium to approximately 2.3 g/d.

- Based on hyperphosphatemia, adjust dietary phosphorus intake, including phosphorus additives, to reduce phosphorus within normal range. Confirm patient is taking phosphorus binders with meals.
- To prevent undesirable weight gain while maintaining dry weight, limit dietary calories to approximately 1,600 kcal/d. (Patient will receive an additional 595 kcal/d from PD exchanges.)
- To replete protein stores in the context of peritonitis, provide approximately 94 g protein per day. Reevaluate adequacy of estimated protein needs at nutrition follow-up.

Nutrition Intervention: Education

Explain to the patient the nutrition modifications needed to reduce fluid and sodium intake due to the presence of edema and hyponatremia.

Explain to the patient the nutrition modifications needed to reduce dietary phosphorus. Help the patient identify different methods to control nausea symptoms, such as switching to a carbonated beverage that is *not* cola to reduce phosphorus intake and eating a moderate amount of low-sodium crackers.

Explain to the patient that she is absorbing additional calories from the peritoneal dialysate and that intake of oral calories will need to be adjusted accordingly to prevent excessive weight gain.

Explain to the patient that her protein needs have increased because of peritonitis, while also educating her about the need to keep her phosphorus intake as low as possible.

Explain findings from laboratory tests and teach the patient how she can adjust her diet in accordance with laboratory results.

Nutrition Intervention: Counseling

Use motivational interviewing to determine how well the patient has accepted her diagnosis and her ability to recognize the changes needed in her diet.

Use motivational interviewing techniques to assure the patient that she can exercise her freedom of choice about how to use information that is provided regarding outcomes (eg, laboratory values) and diet.

References

1. Academy of Nutrition and Dietetics. *Abridged Nutrition Care Process Terminology (NCPT) Reference Manual: Standardized Terminology for the Nutrition Care Process*. Academy of Nutrition and Dietetics; 2018.
2. Academy of Nutrition and Dietetics. Electronic Nutrition Care Process Terminology (eNCPT). Accessed November 29, 2022. www.ncpro.org
3. Ikizler TA, Burrowes JD, Byham-Gray LD, et al. KDOQI clinical practice guideline for nutrition in CKD: 2020 update. *J Kidney Dis*. 2020;76(3 suppl 1):S1-S107. doi:10.1053/j.ajkd.2020.05.006
4. Academy of Nutrition and Dietetics Evidence Analysis Library. Chronic kidney disease (CKD) guideline. 2010. Accessed August 11, 2022. www.andeal.org/topic.cfm?cat=3927&highlight=kidney&home=1
5. Kidney Disease Outcomes Quality Initiative, National Kidney Foundation. Clinical practice guidelines for nutrition in chronic renal failure. *Am J Kidney Dis*. 2000;35(6 suppl 2):S17-S104. doi:10.1053/ajkd.2000.v35.aajkd03517
6. Kidney Disease Outcomes Quality Initiative Workgroup. K/DOQI clinical practice guidelines for cardiovascular disease in dialysis patients. *Am J Kidney Dis*. 2005;45(4 suppl 3):S1-S153.

7. Kidney Disease Outcomes Quality Initiative. KDOQI clinical practice guidelines and clinical practice recommendations for diabetes and chronic kidney disease. *Am J Kidney Dis*. 2007;49(2 Suppl 2):S12-S154. doi:10.1053/j.ajkd.2006.12.005

8. Phillips S, Gonyea J, eds. *Clinical Guide to Nutrition Care in Kidney Disease*. 3rd ed. Academy of Nutrition and Dietetics; 2022.

9. McCann L. *Pocket Guide to Nutrition Assessment of the Patient with Kidney Disease*. 6th ed. National Kidney Foundation; 2021.

10. US Department of Agriculture. *Food Safety: A Need-to-Know Guide for Those at Risk*. Updated 2020. Accessed August 30, 2022. www.fsis.usda.gov/sites/default/files/media_file/2021-04/at-risk-booklet.pdf

11. Franz MJ, Boucher JL, Pereia RF. *Pocket Guide to Lipid Disorders, Hypertension, Diabetes, and Weight Management*. 2nd ed. Academy of Nutrition and Dietetics; 2017.

12. VanWormer JJ, Boucher JL. The 5 A's: behavior change counseling in the context of brief clinical encounters. *On the Cutting Edge*. 2003;24(4):24-26.

13. VanWormer JJ, Boucher JL. Motivational interviewing and diabetes education: fostering commitment to change. *On the Cutting Edge*. 2003;24(4):14-16.

14. VanWormer JJ, Boucher JL. Motivational interviewing and diet modification: a review of the evidence. *Diabetes Educ*. 2004;30:404-419. doi:10.1177/014572170403000309

15. Prochaska JO, Velicer WF. The transtheoretical model of health behavior change. *Am J Health Promot*. 1997;12(1):38-48. doi:10.4278/0890-1171-12.1.38

16. Klein S, Burke LE, Bray GA, et al. Clinical implications of obesity with specific focus on cardiovascular disease: a statement for professionals from the American Heart Association Council on Nutrition, Physical Activity, and Metabolism: endorsed by the American College of Cardiology Foundation. *Circulation*. 2004;110(18):2952-2967. doi:10.1161/01.CIR.0000145546.97738.1E

17. Artinian NT, Fletcher GF, Mozaffarian D, et al. Interventions to promote physical activity and dietary lifestyle changes for cardiovascular risk factor reduction in adults: a scientific statement from the American Heart Association. *Circulation*. 2010;122(4):406-441. doi:10.1161/CIR.0b013e3181e8edf1

CHAPTER 6

Nutrition Monitoring and Evaluation

The final step in the Nutrition Care Process (NCP) is monitoring, measuring, and evaluating changes in nutrition care indicators to determine whether a patient is meeting the agreed-upon nutrition goals or outcomes. In chronic kidney disease (CKD), a patient's progress toward specific reference standards must be determined as part of monitoring and evaluation.[1,2]

Outcomes and acceptable goals may change as a patient moves from one stage of CKD to the next or as treatment modalities change (eg, medical management, hemodialysis [HD], peritoneal dialysis [PD], or transplantation). Following is a list of potential outcomes that may be used for monitoring the patient with CKD[1]:

- food- and nutrition-related history: changes in energy, fluid, macronutrient, and micronutrient intake; food and nutrition knowledge, beliefs, and attitudes; estimated energy, macronutrient, fluid and micronutrient needs
- changes in biochemical data, medical tests, and procedures
- changes in anthropometric measurements
- nutrition focused physical findings

When accepted evidence-based standards are used, monitoring and evaluation of the aforementioned factors can determine the effectiveness of medical nutrition therapy in adults who have CKD and those who are post–kidney transplant.

Monitoring and Evaluation Recommendations

Specific nutrition monitoring and evaluation recommendations for patients with CKD can be found in the 2020 update of the Kidney Disease Outcomes Quality Initiative (KDOQI) clinical practice guideline for nutrition in CKD from the National Kidney Foundation and the Academy of Nutrition and Dietetics.[3] See Box 6.1 for a summary of these recommendations.[3] For nutrition monitoring and evaluation, the registered dietitian nutritionist (RDN) should follow up with individuals with CKD at regular intervals. Box 2.7 on page 33 lists biochemical parameters that may be monitored in CKD, with suggestions about why each parameter is utilized. Box 6.2 on page 172 suggests how often certain parameters may be evaluated in patients with CKD who are on dialysis.[3]

Documentation of Nutrition Care

Documentation of nutrition care in the patient's medical record is the primary way of communicating the nutrition goals and expected outcomes to the health care team. The documentation should be complete, concise, and in the format and style that is determined by facility or practice policy.

There are many different charting formats that can be used. Within the Nutrition Care Process and Terminology (NCPT), a documentation model that follows the four steps of the NCP has been developed using the ADIME (assessment, diagnosis, intervention, and monitoring and evaluation) format. If an electronic health record is being used, building standardized language into the health record will facilitate data collection and lead to a standardized nutrition data set. In 2009, the American Dietetic Association (now the Academy of Nutrition and Dietetics) published a white paper to address the need for a nutrition data set. This paper outlines the nutrition data set elements needed in an electronic medical record: height and weight, BMI, waist circumference, blood pressure, fasting lipoprotein profile, C-reactive protein, serum albumin, lifestyle habits assessment, level of physical fitness, and referral to the RDN.[4] Key elements to consider when charting each of the NCP steps can be found in Box 6.3 on page 173.[5]

BOX 6.1 Nutrition Monitoring and Evaluation Recommendations[3]

The registered dietitian nutritionist (RDN) should, at least annually or when indicated by nutrition screening or referral, monitor and evaluate various parameters in adults with chronic kidney disease (CKD), including post–kidney transplant, related to the following:

- Appetite
- History of dietary intake
- Body weight
- BMI
- Biochemical data
  - Glycemic control
  - Protein-energy malnutrition
  - Inflammation
  - Kidney function
  - Mineral and bone disorders
  - Anemia
  - Dyslipidemia
  - Electrolyte disorders
  - Others as appropriate
- Anthropometric measurements
- Nutrition focused physical findings
- Effectiveness of medical nutrition therapy
- Food and nutrient intake (eg, diet history, diet experience, and intake of calcium, phosphorus, and others, as appropriate) and intake of macronutrients and micronutrients such as energy, protein, sodium, and potassium
- Medication (prescription and over the counter), dietary supplement (vitamin, minerals, protein, etc), and herbal or botanical supplement use
- Knowledge, beliefs, or attitudes (eg, readiness to change nutrition and lifestyle behaviors)
- Behavior
- Factors affecting access to food and food- and nutrition-related supplies (eg, safe food and meal availability)

> **BOX 6.2   Recommended Measures for Monitoring Nutritional Status of Patients on Maintenance Dialysis Annually or When Status Change Indicates[3,a]**
>
> ### Category 1: Routine measurements[b]
>
> Predialysis or stabilized serum albumin: Measure at least once a month.
>
> Percentage of usual post–hemodialysis (HD) or post–peritoneal dialysis (PD) drain body weight: Measure at least once a month.
>
> Subjective global assessment: Measure at least every 4 months.
>
> Dietary interview and/or diary: Measure at least every 6 months.
>
> Normalized protein nitrogen appearance: Measure at least every 6 months.
>
> ### Category 2: Measures to confirm or extend the data from the category 1 measurements
>
> Predialysis or stabilized serum prealbumin: Measure at least monthly in HD; at least every 3 to 4 months in PD.
>
> Skinfold thickness: Measure as needed.
>
> Midarm muscle area, circumference, or diameter: Measure as needed.
>
> Dual energy x-ray absorptiometry: Measure as needed.
>
> ### Category 3: Other clinically useful measures
>
> **Note:** *Low values in this category might suggest the need for more rigorous examination of protein-energy nutritional status. Measure as needed.*
>
> Predialysis or stabilized serum creatinine
>
> Predialysis or stabilized serum urea nitrogen
>
> Predialysis or stabilized serum cholesterol
>
> Creatinine index

[a] The Centers for Medicare and Medicaid Services have established a Measures Assessment Tool (MAT), which outlines specific time frames for nutrition monitoring for patients on dialysis (www.cms.gov/Medicare/Provider-Enrollment-and-Certification/GuidanceforLawsAndRegulations/Dialysis.html). According to MAT, the following should be monitored monthly: albumin, body weight, calcium, and phosphorus. Hemoglobin should also be monitored monthly in patients who are not taking an erythropoiesis-stimulating agent (ESA) and those taking an ESA who are stable. Monitor hemoglobin weekly in patients taking an ESA who are not stable. Parathyroid hormone should be monitored every 3 months, and other nutritional parameters should be monitored as needed.

[b] These measurements should be performed routinely in all patients.

BOX 6.3 Key Nutrition Care Process–Related Charting Elements for Medical Records

Nutrition assessment
Date and time of assessment

Pertinent data collected and comparisons with standards (eg, food and nutrition history, biochemical data, anthropometric measurements, patient history, medical nutrition therapy use, and supplement use)

Patient's readiness to learn, food- and nutrition-related knowledge, and potential for change

Physical activity history and goals

Reason for discontinuation of nutrition therapy, if applicable

Nutrition diagnosis
Date and time

Concise written statement of nutrition diagnosis/diagnoses written in the PES (problem, etiology, signs and symptoms) format

If there is no existing nutrition problem, state "no nutrition diagnosis at this time"

Nutrition intervention
Date and time

Specific treatment goals and expected outcomes

Recommended nutrition prescription and individualized nutrition intervention

Any adjustments to plan and justification

Patient's attitude regarding recommendations

Changes in patient's attitude regarding recommendations

Changes in patient's level of understanding and food-related behaviors

Referrals made and resources used

Any other information relevant to providing care and monitoring progress over time

Plans for follow-up and frequency

Continued on next page

> **BOX 6.3 Key Nutrition Care Process–Related Charting Elements for Medical Records (cont.)**
>
> ### Nutrition Monitoring and Evaluation
> Date and time
>
> Specific nutrition outcome indicators and results relevant to the nutrition diagnosis and intervention plans and goals, compared with previous status or reference goals
>
> Progress toward nutrition intervention goals
>
> Factors facilitating or hindering progress
>
> Other positive or negative outcomes
>
> Future plans for nutrition care, monitoring, and follow-up or discharge

Adapted with permission from Franz MJ, Boucher JL, Pereira RF. *Pocket Guide to Lipid Disorders, Hypertension, Diabetes, and Weight Management*. 2nd ed. Academy of Nutrition and Dietetics; 2017.

Case Study

Nutrition Care Process

Step 4: Nutrition Monitoring and Evaluation

> This chapter adds the monitoring and evaluation piece of the NCP to information captured in the assessment presented in Chapter 2, development of the diagnosis presented in Chapter 3, and planning and implementation of the nutrition intervention presented in Chapters 4 and 5. New information is set off from the previous material in white. In this final installment, outcome indicators are described using the standardized language of the NCP; criteria to evaluate outcomes are also listed (see Box at the end of the full case study).

A 56-year-old female individual with CKD stage 5D on peritoneal dialysis is admitted to the hospital.

Nutrition Assessment

Food/Nutrition-Related History

Food Intake
Patient consumes traditional Cambodian foods and follows traditional Cambodian meal patterns, including rice, stir-fried vegetables, and small amounts of fish, poultry, and beef. Uses fish sauce frequently. Has been consuming increased amounts of cola soft drinks to ease nausea.

Medications
HMG-CoA reductase inhibitor (statin), renal multivitamin, calcium carbonate and sevelamer with meals, calcitriol, ferrous sulfate, insulin

aspart with meals, isoniazid, vitamin B6, and lansoprazole. Has missed a few days of taking medications because of current condition.

Food and Nutrition Knowledge/Skill
Family is aware of low phosphorus and low potassium foods; is very involved.

Physical activity
Sedentary

Anthropometric Measurements

Body Composition, Growth, and Weight History

Height
150 cm (59 in)

Admit weight
74.5 kg (164 lb)

Estimated dry weight (EDW)
72 kg (has been stable)

BMI (using EDW)
32

Frame size
Medium

Ideal body weight (IBW)
62 kg; 116% IBW

Biochemical Data, Medical Tests, and Procedures

Electrolyte and renal profile
See laboratory data table.

Nutritional anemia profile
See laboratory data table.

Urine output
500 mL/24 h

Laboratory Data for Nutrition Assessment of Patient[3]		
Laboratory test	Reference range	Patient result
Potassium, mmol/L	Normal: 3.4-5 Peritoneal dialysis (PD)[a]: 3.5-5.5	5.4
Blood urea nitrogen, mg/dL	Normal: 6-20 PD: >60	58
Creatinine, mg/dL	Normal: 0.7-1.3 PD: not defined	11
Glucose, mg/dL	Normal (fasting): 60-99	92
Calcium, mg/dL	Normal: 8.6-10.2	8.8
Phosphorus, mg/dL	Normal: 2.4-4.7 PD: 3.5-5.5	5.7
Albumin, g/dL	Normal: 3.5-4.7 PD: >3.5	1.6
Hemoglobin, g/dL	Normal: 13.5-17.5 PD: 10-12	9
Capillary blood glucose, mg/dL	Normal: <150	120-250
Sodium, mmol/L	Normal: 134-143	129

[a] Reference range for patients on peritoneal dialysis.

Nutrition Focused Physical Findings

- Overall appearance: abrasions on arms and neck from scratching
- Obese with central adiposity
- Bilateral ankle edema and edema of eyelid

- Diarrhea, nausea, and vomiting
- Pale conjunctiva
- Koilonychia (spoon-shaped nails)

Patient History

Personal data: Patient is 56-year-old female individual, does not speak English; children are fluent in English and are very involved and supportive.

Patient or family nutrition-oriented medical/health history: ESRD due to hypertension. History includes type 2 diabetes. Admitted to the hospital with peritonitis, pain, nausea, vomiting, and fever. Third episode of peritonitis in 2 months. Latent tuberculosis.

Treatment/therapy: Peritoneal dialysis with five exchanges per day, each 2 L 2.5% dextrose. Type 2 diabetes mellitus managed with insulin; capillary blood glucose usually less than 250 mg/dL.

Nutrition Diagnosis

Intake Domain

Nutrition Diagnosis

Excessive mineral intake (sodium)

Sample PES Statement

Excessive sodium intake related to cultural food patterns as evidenced by diet recall revealing frequent use of fish sauce as well as presence of ankle and orbital edema.

Clinical Domain

Nutrition Diagnosis

Altered nutrition-related laboratory values (serum phosphorus and albumin)

Sample PES Statements

- Altered nutrition-related laboratory values (serum phosphorus) related to missed binder doses as evidenced by patient report and serum phosphorus value of 5.7 mg/dL.
- Altered nutrition-related laboratory values (serum albumin) related to altered nutrient utilization in inflammatory state as evidenced by serum albumin of 1.6 g/dL in a patient with acute peritonitis.

Behavioral-Environmental Domain

Nutrition Diagnosis

Limited adherence to nutrition-related recommendations

Sample PES Statement

Limited adherence to nutrition-related recommendations related to the use of high-phosphorus soft drinks to treat gastrointestinal symptoms as evidenced by patient reports of drinking cola beverages during episodes of nausea.

Nutrition Intervention

Peritoneal Dialysis Regimen

Patient receives PD with five exchanges per day, each 2 L 2.5% dextrose.

Note: 2.5% dextrose provides 25 g dextrose/L (see Table 4.7 on page 111 for additional information on dextrose contributions).

Calculate calories from daily PD exchanges as follows:

$$2 \text{ L per exchange} \times (25 \text{ g dextrose/L}) = 50 \text{ g dextrose per PD exchange}$$

$$(50 \text{ g dextrose per PD exchange}) \times (5 \text{ PD exchanges/d}) = 250 \text{ g dextrose/d}$$

$$(250 \text{ g dextrose/d}) \times (3.4 \text{ kcal/g dextrose}) = 850 \text{ kcal/d}$$

$$(850 \text{ kcal/d}) \times 70\% \text{ absorption} = 595 \text{ kcal/d from PD exchanges}$$

Calculating Energy and Protein Needs

Note: Calculation uses dry weight
Energy needs:

$$72 \text{ kg} \times 25 \text{ to } 30 \text{ kcal/kg/d} = 1,800 \text{ to } 2,160 \text{ kcal/d}$$

Subtract 595 kcal provided by PD regimen = 1,205 to 1,565 kcal/d

Protein needs (increased due to peritonitis):

$$72 \text{ kg} \times 1.3 \text{ g/kg/d} = 94 \text{ g/d}$$

Daily Nutrition Prescription for Patient Undergoing Peritoneal Dialysis

Other elements of the nutrition prescription are as follows:
- Based on the patient's past medical history and calculated macronutrient and micronutrient needs, suggest a renal, carbohydrate-controlled diet adjusted to cultural food preferences as permissible within renal and diabetic requirements.
- Based on urine output of 500 mL/24 h and edema/hyponatremia, suggest limiting dietary fluid intake to 1,000 mL/d.
- Based on edema/hyponatremia, suggest limiting dietary sodium to approximately 2.3 g/d.
- Based on hyperphosphatemia, adjust dietary phosphorus intake, including phosphorus additives, to reduce phosphorus within normal range. Confirm patient is taking phosphorus binders with meals.

- To prevent undesirable weight gain while maintaining dry weight, limit dietary calories to approximately 1,600 kcal/d. (Patient will receive an additional 595 kcal/d from PD exchanges.)
- To replete protein stores in the context of peritonitis, provide approximately 94 g protein per day. Reevaluate adequacy of estimated protein needs at nutrition follow-up.

Nutrition Intervention (Education)

Explain to the patient the nutrition modifications needed to reduce fluid and sodium intake due to the presence of edema and hyponatremia.

Explain to the patient the nutrition modifications needed to reduce dietary phosphorus. Help the patient identify different methods to control nausea symptoms, such as switching to a carbonated beverage that is *not* cola to reduce phosphorus intake and eating a moderate amount of low-sodium crackers.

Explain to the patient that she is absorbing additional calories from the peritoneal dialysate, and that intake of oral calories will need to be adjusted accordingly to prevent excessive weight gain.

Explain to the patient that her protein needs have increased because of peritonitis, while also educating her about the need to keep her phosphorus intake as low as possible.

Explain findings from laboratory tests and teach the patient how she can adjust her diet in accordance with laboratory results.

Nutrition Intervention (Counseling)

Use motivational interviewing to determine how well the patient has accepted her diagnosis and her ability to recognize the changes needed in her diet.

Use motivational interviewing techniques to assure the patient that she can exercise her freedom of choice about how to use information that is provided regarding outcomes (eg, laboratory values) and diet.

Nutrition Monitoring and Evaluation

See the box below for outcome indicators described using the standardized language of the NCP; criteria to evaluate outcomes are also listed.

Outcome indicator	Criterion
Food- and nutrition-related history	
Protein intake	Patient can explain how peritonitis affects protein needs; will identify foods to add 10 to 14 g protein per day.
Vitamin intake	Patient takes renal-specific multivitamin.
Mineral intake—sodium	Patient uses less fish sauce and less of other high-sodium sauces.
Mineral intake—phosphorus	Patient decreases use of cola to treat nausea.
Beliefs and attitudes	Patient understands the severity of risk to her health.
Biochemical data, medical tests, and procedures	
Nutritional anemia profile	Team will evaluate iron stores and adjust treatment as appropriate.
Electrolyte and renal profile	Patient can explain at least one of the monthly tests and how her diet can be adjusted in context of results.
Anthropometric measurements	
Weight change	Patient will achieve a gradual decrease in BMI to <30.
Nutrition focused physical findings	
Extremities, muscles, bones Head and eyes	Patient has less edema in legs and face.

References

1. Academy of Nutrition and Dietetics. *Abridged Nutrition Care Process Terminology (NCPT) Reference Manual: Standardized Terminology for the Nutrition Care Process*. Academy of Nutrition and Dietetics; 2018.
2. Academy of Nutrition and Dietetics. Electronic Nutrition Care Process Terminology (eNCPT). Accessed November 29, 2022. www.ncpro.org
3. Ikizler TA, Burrowes JD, Byham-Gray LD, et al. KDOQI clinical practice guideline for nutrition in CKD: 2020 update. *J Kidney Dis*. 2020;76(3 suppl 1):S1-S107. doi:10.1053/j.ajkd.2020.05.006
4. Peregrin T. Personal and electronic health records: sharing nutrition information across the health care community. *J Am Diet Assoc*. 2009;109(12):1988-1991. doi:10.1016/j.jada.2009.10.022
5. Franz MJ, Boucher JL, Pereira RF. *Pocket Guide to Lipid Disorders, Hypertension, Diabetes, and Weight Management*. Academy of Nutrition and Dietetics; 2017.

APPENDIX

Commonly Prescribed Renal-Specific Vitamins[a]

Commonly Prescribed Renal-Specific Vitamins[a]

Product	Folic acid, mg	Thiamin (B1), mg	Riboflavin (B2), mg	Niacin (B3), mg	Pantothenic acid (B5), mg	Pyridoxine (B6), mg	Cobalamin (B12), mcg	Biotin, mcg	Vitamin C, mg	Vitamin D3, IU	Vitamin E, IU	Zinc, mg	Copper, mg	Selenium, mcg
Prescription														
Dialyvite Rx[b]	1	1.5	1.7	20	10	10	6	300	100	0	0	0	0	0
Dialyvite With Zinc Rx[b]	1	1.5	1.7	20	10	10	6	300	100	0	0	50	0	0
Dialyvite 3000[b]	3	1.5	1.7	20	10	25	1	300	100	0	30	15	0	70
Dialyvite 5000[b]	5	1.5	1.7	20	10	50	2	300	100	0	30	25	0	70
Dialyvite Supreme D Rx[b]	3	1.5	1.7	20	10	25	1	300	100	2,000	30	15	0	70
Folbee Plus[c]	5	1.5	1.5	20	10	50	1	300	60	0	0	0	0	0
Folbee Plus CZ[c]	5	1.5	1.7	20	10	50	2	300	60	0	0	25	1.5	0
Nephrocap[d]	1	1.5	1.7	20	5	10	6	150	100	0	0	0	0	0
Nephronex[e]	0.9	1.5	1.7	20	10	10	10	300	60	0	0	0	0	0
NephPlex Rx[f]	1	1.5	1.7	20	10	10	6	300	60	0	0	12.5	0	0
RenaCaps[g]	1	1.5	1.7	20	5	10	6	150	10	0	0	0	0	0
Vital-D Rx[c]	1	1.5	1.7	20	10	10	6	300	60	2,000	35	12.5	0	70
Nephro-Vite Rx[h]	1	1.5	1.7	20	10	10	6	300	60	0	0	0	0	0
Vital-D Rx[i]	1	1.5	1.7	20	10	10	6	300	60	1,750	0	12.5	0	70
Over the counter														
Dialyvite 800[b]	0.8	1.5	1.7	20	10	10	6	300	60	0	0	0	0	0
Dialyvite 800 With Iron[b]	0.8	1.5	1.7	20	10	10	6	300	60	0	0	0	0	0
Dialyvite 800 With Zinc[b]	0.8	1.5	1.7	20	10	10	6	300	60	0	0	50	0	0

Continued on next page

Product	Folic acid, mg	Thiamin (B1), mg	Riboflavin (B2), mg	Niacin (B3), mg	Pantothenic acid (B5), mg	Pyridoxine (B6), mg	Cobalamin (B12), mcg	Biotin, mcg	Vitamin C, mg	Vitamin D3, IU	Vitamin E, IU	Zinc, mg	Copper, mg	Selenium, mcg
Dialyvite 800 With Zinc 15[b]	0.8	1.5	1.7	20	10	10	6	300	60	0	0	15	0	0
Dialyvite 800/Ultra D[b]	0.8	1.5	1.7	20	10	10	6	300	60	2,000	30	15	0	70
Dialyvite 800 Plus D Chewable[b]	0.8	1.5	1.7	20	10	10	6	300	60	2,000	0	0	0	0
Dialyvite 800 Chewable[b]	0.8	1.5	1.7	20	10	10	6	300	60	0	0	0	0	0
Dialyvite 800 Liquid[b]	0.8	1.5	1.7	20	10	10	6	300	60	0	0	0	0	0
Nephronex Liquid[c]	0.9	1.5	1.7	20	10	10	10	300	60	0	0	0	0	0
Nephro Vite[k]	0.8	1.5	1.7	20	10	10	6	300	60	0	0	0	0	0
ProRenal+D[f]	0.8	1.5	2	20	5	10	2.4	30	60	1,000	0	8	0.9	55
RenalTab[g]	1	1.5	1.7	20	10	10	6	300	60	0	0	0	0	0
RenalTab Zn[g]	1	1.5	1.7	20	10	10	6	300	60	0	0	15	0	0
RenalTab Zn + D[g]	1	1.5	1.7	20	10	10	6	300	60	1,000	0	15	0	0
RenaPlex[i]	0.8	1.5	1.7	20	10	10	6	300	60	0	0	0	0	0
RenaPlex-D[i]	0.8	1.5	1.7	20	10	10	6	300	60	2,000	35	12.5	0	70
Rena-Vite[a]	0.8	1.5	1.7	20	10	10	6	300	60	0	0	0	0	0

[a] This list is not all-inclusive of renal vitamins, and contents are subject to change. Check manufacturer websites and product labeling for up-to-date information.

[b–k] Manufacturers are as follows: [b] Dialyvite Renal Products (a division of Hillestad Pharmaceuticals USA Inc). Woodruff, WI 54568 (www.dialyvite.net); [c] Breckenridge Pharmaceuticals, Berlin, CT 06037 (www.bpirx.com); [d] Bausch Health, Laval, Quebec, Canada (www.bauschhealth.com); [e] Llorens Pharmaceuticals, Miami, FL 33166 (www.llorenspharm.com); [f] Nephro-Tech, Shawnee, KS 66203 (www.nephrotech.com); [g] Nnodum Pharmaceuticals, Cincinnati, OH 45240 (www.zikspain.com); [h] Allergan Pharmaceutical Morristown, NJ 07960 (www.allergan.com); [i] Nephroceuticals, Beavercreek, OH 54352 (http://myprorenal.com); [j] Renalab Inc. Templeton, CA 93465 (http://renalab.net); [k] Cypress Pharmaceutical Inc. Morristown, NJ 07960.

Continuing Professional Education

The second edition of the *Academy of Nutrition and Dietetics Pocket Guide to Chronic Kidney Disease and the Nutrition Care Process* offers readers 2 hours of Continuing Professional Education (CPE) credit expiring December, 31, 2025. Readers may earn credit by completing the interactive quiz at: https://publications.webauthor.com/PG_CKD_NCP2e

Index

Page numbers followed by *f* indicate figures, page number followed by *t* indicates tables, and page numbers followed by *b* indicate boxes.

AA. *See* amino acids (AA)
Abridged Nutrition Care Process Terminology (NCPT) Reference Manual, 1, 15, 62, 138, 152
Academy of Nutrition and Dietetics, 1, 140*b*
Academy of Nutrition and Dietetics Pocket Guide to Lipid Disorders, Hypertension, Diabetes, and Weight Management, 152
acarbose, 27*b*
access etiology, 63
acebutolol (Sectral), 20*b*
Aceon. *See* perindopril (Aceon)
acetohexamide, 27*b*
acid-base balance, 84, 102
acid load, 84, 102
acute kidney injury, 47*b*
Adalat CC. *See* long-acting nifedipine (Adalat CC, Procardia XL)
ADIME nutrition assessment, 4*b*
adipose, 43
adjusted body weight, 45*b*–46*b*
Advise step, in nutrition counseling, 158
Agree step, in nutrition counseling, 158–159
albumin, 37*b*, 127, 179
alcohol, 30*b*
Aldactone. *See* spironolactone (Aldactone, CaroSpir)
Aldomet. *See* methyldopa (Aldomet)
Aldosterone receptor blockers, 19*b*
alkaline phosphatase, 37*b*, 43*b*
Alpha1 blockers, 20*b*, 22*b*

Alpha-Glucosidase Inhibitors, 27*b*
Altace. *See* ramipril (Altace)
aluminum, 37*b*, 105
  hydroxide, 22*b*, 86
American Academy of Kidney Patients, 140*b*
American Society for Parenteral and Enteral Nutrition (ASPEN), 2, 110
American Society of Nephrology (ASN), 3
amiloride (Midamor), 19*b*
amino acids (AA), 88*t*, 89*b*, 109*b*
  dialysate, 106, 110
  oral, 77*t*
  supplementation, 110
amlodipine (Norvasc), 21*b*
Amphojel, 22*b*
amputation, 46*b*
Amylin Analogs, 28*b*
anemia, 2, 122
  assessment, 35*b*
  iron-deficiency, 81, 119
angiotensin-converting enzyme inhibitors, 20*b*
angiotensin II receptor blockers/antagonists, 21*b*
antacids, 30*b*, 86
anthropometric measurements, 32–34, 33*b*–34*b*, 66, 124–125, 176
antibiotics, 30*b*
anticoagulants, 30*b*, 116*b*, 119
anticonvulsants, 30*b*
antigout medications, 30*b*
antihypertensives, 19*b*–22*b*

antiproliferative medications, 30*b*
antithymocyte globulin (ATG), 150*b*
appetite
  enhanced, 149*b*
  stimulants, 143, 144*b*
Apresoline. *See* hydralazine (Apresoline)
Arrange step, in nutrition counseling, 159
arteriovenous (AV) grafts, 98*b*
Ask step, in nutrition counseling, 153, 153*b*–154*b*
ASN. *See* American Society of Nephrology (ASN)
ASPEN. *See* American Society for Parenteral and Enteral Nutrition (ASPEN)
Assess step, in nutrition counseling, 154–155, 155*b*–158*b*
Atacand. *See* candesartan (Atacand)
atenolol (Tenormin), 20*b*
ATG. *See* antithymocyte globulin (ATG)
Atorvastatin, 29*b*
Auryxia, 24*b*
Avapro. *See* irbesartan (Avapro)
AV grafts. *See* arteriovenous (AV) grafts
azathioprine (Imuran), 30*b*, 149*b*

basiliximab (Simulect), 150*b*
B-complex vitamin, 101, 116*b*, 120
behavioral-environmental findings, 55, 61*b*–62*b*, 69, 127–128, 179
behavior etiology, 63
beliefs-attitudes etiology, 62–63
benazepril (Lotensin), 20*b*
Beneprotein, 136*b*
Benicar. *See* olmesartan (Benicar)
Beta blockers, 20*b*
betaxolol (Kerlone), 20*b*
bicarbonate, 102, 110
Biguanides, 28*b*
bile acid sequestrants, 29*b*
bioactive substances, 71*b*, 133
biochemical data, 34, 35*b*–42*b*, 66–68, 125–126, 162–163, 176–178
biotin, 91*b*, 100*b*, 185–186
bisoprolol (Zebeta), 20*b*
Blocadren. *See* timolol (Blocadren)
blood glucose levels, 95–96, 109*b*, 110, 115*b*

blood pressure, 2, 75, 102, 112*b*, 120
blood urea nitrogen, 38*b*
BMI classification, 32–33, 33*b*, 66
body weight (BW), 32, 45*b*–46*b*, 60*b*, 75, 93*b*
bone(s)
  disease, metabolic, 43*b*
  health, 35*b*
  integrity, 85
Boost, 136*b*, 137*b*
bumetanide (Bumex), 19*b*
Bumex. *See* bumetanide (Bumex)
burns, 47*b*
BW. *See* body weight (BW)

Ca. *See* calcium (Ca); minerals
Calan. *See* immediate-release verapamil (Calan, Isoptin)
Calan SR. *See* long-acting verapamil (Calan SR, Isoptin SR)
calcidiol, 43*b*
calcineurin inhibitors, 31*b*, 121
Calcitriol, 124
calcium (Ca), 71*b*. *See also* minerals
calcium channel blockers, 21*b*
calorie boosters, 145*t*
Calphron, 23*b*
candesartan (Atacand), 21*b*
Capoten. *See* captopril (Capoten)
captopril (Capoten), 20*b*
carbohydrate, 72*t*, 88*t*, 93*b*, 114*b*–115*b*
  intake, 78, 144–146, 145*t*, 146*b*
  prescription, 78–79, 96–97, 118
cardiac arrhythmia, 103
cardiac function, 85, 103
cardiomyopathy, 87, 106
cardiovascular disease, 97, 118
cardiovascular events, 97*b*
Cardizem CD. *See* extended-release diltiazem (Cardizem CD, Dilacor XR, Tiazac, Cardizem LA)
Cardizem LA. *See* extended-release diltiazem (Cardizem CD, Dilacor XR, Tiazac, Cardizem LA)
Cardura. *See* doxazosin (Cardura)
Carnation Breakfast Essentials, 136*b*
CaroSpir. *See* spironolactone (Aldactone, CaroSpir)
carvedilol (Coreg), 20*b*

Catapres. *See* clonidine (Catapres)
Catapres-TTS. *See* clonidine patch (Catapres-TTS)
Cellcept. *See* mycophenolate mofetil (Cellcept, RS-61443)
Centers for Medicare and Medicaid Services, U.S. (CMS), 2
Central Alpha2 Agonists, 22*b*
centrally acting drugs, 22*b*
CfC. *See* Conditions for Coverage
chloride, 90*b*
chlorothiazide (Diuril), 19*b*
Chlorpropamide, 27*b*
cholecalciferol (vitamin D3), 80–81, 116*b*, 119, 185–186
cholesterol, 71*b*, 73*t*
cholestyramine, 29*b*
chromium, 91*b*
chronic kidney disease (CKD), 1, 47*b*, 56, 71, 133, 169
  anemia in, 2
  blood pressure in, 2
  diabetes and, 146*b*
  dyslipidemia in, 2
  evaluation and management of, 2
  formulas, 138*b*
  management of, 15
  MNT and, 2–10, 4*b*, 5*t*, 7*b*, 9*b*
  nutrition prescription for, 71*b*
  self-management, 146*b*
  stages of, 3*t*, 3–4, 8–10, 9*b*
Chronic Kidney Disease Epidemiology Collaboration (CKD-EPI), 3
chronic kidney disease-mineral and bone disorder (CKD-MBD), 2, 75, 117
Citracal, 24*b*
citric acid, 102
CKD. *See* chronic kidney disease (CKD)
CKD-EPI. *See* Chronic Kidney Disease Epidemiology Collaboration (CKD-EPI)
CKD-MBD. *See* chronic kidney disease-mineral and bone disorder (CKD-MBD)
clinical domain, 68, 178
Clinical Guide to Nutrition Care in Kidney Disease, 140*b*
clonidine (Catapres), 22*b*
clonidine patch (Catapres-TTS), 22*b*

CMS. *See* Centers for Medicare and Medicaid Services, U.S. (CMS)
cobalamin (vitamin B12), 83*b*, 100*b*, 185–186
colesevelam, 29*b*
colestipol, 29*b*
Conditions for Coverage (CfC), 2, 9*b*
continuous renal replacement therapy (CRRT), 90*b*
conventional home hemodialysis, 111
copper, 91*b*, 185–186
  deficiency, 87, 105
Coreg. *See* carvedilol (Coreg)
Corgard. *See* nadolol (Corgard)
corticosteroids, 31*b*, 149*b*, 150*b*
Covera HS. *See* extended-release verapamil hydrochloride (Covera HS, Verelan PM)
COVID-19 pandemic, Medicare and, 6
Cozaar. *See* losartan (Cozaar)
creatinine (Cr), 27*b*, 38*b*
CRRT. *See* continuous renal replacement therapy (CRRT)
cultural etiology, 63
Cushingoid appearance, 43, 149*b*
cyanocobalamin (vitamin B12), 42*b*, 81, 91*b*, 101, 116*b*, 120
Cycloserine, 30*b*
cyclosporine A (Sandimmune, Neoral), 31*b*, 149*b*
cystatin C, 3

daclizumab (Zenapax), 150*b*
DASH diet. *See* Dietary Approaches to Stop Hypertension (DASH) diet
dermatosis, 87, 106
dextrose, 88*t*, 89*b*, 96, 96*t*, 109*b*, 128
diabetes, 97, 102
  CKD self-management and, 146*b*
  management, 2–
  new-onset, 118
diabetic kidney disease (DKD), 76, 78, 95
diabetic nephropathy, 81
dialysate, 96
  calcium, 103
dialysis, 99
  hemodialysis, 10, 47*b*
  peritoneal, 5
  schedules, 111–112, 111*t*, 112*b*

Dialyvite, 185–186
diet
  counseling, 87–88
  exchanges, 71*b*, 145*t*
  patterns, 74–75, 113, 117
  renal, 96
Dietary Approaches to Stop Hypertension (DASH) diet, 85
Dietary Reference Intakes (DRIs), 114*b*, 119
dihydropyridines, 21*b*
Dilacor XR. *See* extended-release diltiazem (Cardizem CD, Dilacor XR, Tiazac, Cardizem LA)
Diovan. *See* valsartan (Diovan)
Dipeptidyl Peptidase-4 Inhibitors, 28*b*
direct vasodilators, 22*b*
diuretics, 31*b*
Diuril. *See* chlorothiazide (Diuril)
DKD. *See* diabetic kidney disease (DKD)
doxazosin (Cardura), 22*b*
DRIs. *See* Dietary Reference Intakes (DRIs)
dronabinol (Marinol), 144*b*
Dynacirc CR. *See* isradipine (Dynacirc CR)
Dyrenium. *See* torsemide (Dyrenium); triamterene (Dyrenium)
dyslipidemia, 2, 35*b*, 113

edema, 22*b*, 44, 114*b*, 129
edema-free body weight, 46*b*
EDW. *See* estimated dry weight (EDW)
eGFR. *See* estimated glomerular filtration rate (eGFR)
electrolyte(s), 35*b*, 73*t*, 109*b*, 116*b*
  intake, 88
  prescription, 83–87, 102–106, 104*t*, 120–121
elemental formulas, 137*b*
elemental iron, 148*t*
Eliphos, 23*b*
enalapril (Vasotec), 20*b*
encephalopathy, 105
endogenous filtration markers, 3
end-stage kidney disease (ESKD), 76
end-stage renal disease (ESRD), 2, 56
  Medicare regulations for, 5
  risk for, 75

energy, 72*t*, 89*b*, 93*b*, 112*b*, 114*b*–115*b*, 128, 136*b*
  dextrose-based, 96
  intake, 57*b*
  needs, 47*b*, 71*b*
  prescription, 77–78, 95–96, 96*t*, 117
Ensure, 136*b*
enteral formulas, 136*b*
enteral nutrition, 71*b*, 87, 123, 133, 135
  prescription, 88, 107
  tube feeding, 106
eplerenone (Inspra), 19*b*
eprosartan (Teveten), 21*b*
ergocalciferol (vitamin D2), 80–81, 116*b*, 119
erythropoiesis, 122
erythropoiesis-stimulating agent, 105
ESKD. *See* end-stage kidney disease (ESKD)
ESRD. *See* end-stage renal disease (ESRD)
estimated dry weight (EDW), 66
estimated glomerular filtration rate (eGFR), 3–4, 81. *See also* glomerular filtration rate (GFR)
etiology, 55–56
evidence-based practice, 1
exenatide, 28*b*
extended-release diltiazem (Cardizem CD, Dilacor XR, Tiazac, Cardizem LA), 21*b*
extended-release metoprolol (Toprol XL), 20*b*
extended-release verapamil hydrochloride (Covera HS, Verelan PM), 21*b*
ezetimibe, 29*b*
EzFe. *See* iron polysaccharide complex (EzFe, Ferrex 150, Niferex, Niferex-150)

fat, 112*b*, 114*b*–115*b*
  distribution, 71*b*
  emulsions, 89, 89*t*
  intake, 144–146, 145*t*, 146*b*
  prescription, 79, 97, 97*b*–98*b*, 118
fatty acid, 73*t*
FE-40. *See* ferrous gluconate (FE-40, Fergon)

felodipine (Plendil), 21b
fenofibrate, 29b
Feosol. *See* ferrous sulfate (Feosol, Slow Fe)
Fergon. *See* ferrous gluconate (FE-40, Fergon)
Ferrex 150. *See* iron polysaccharide complex (EzFe, Ferrex 150, Niferex, Niferex-150)
ferric citrate, 24b
ferritin, 38b, 39b, 105, 122
Ferro-Sequels. *See* ferrous fumarate (Ferro-Sequels, Hemocyte, Nephro-Fer)
ferrous fumarate (Ferro-Sequels, Hemocyte, Nephro-Fer), 148t
ferrous gluconate (FE-40, Fergon), 148t
ferrous sulfate (Feosol, Slow Fe), 124, 148t
fiber, 71b, 73t
  formulas, 137b
  intake, 144–146, 145t, 146b
Fibric Acid Derivatives, 29b
fish oil, 79, 93b
FK506. *See* tacrolimus (Prograf, FK506)
flaxseed, 93b
fluid(s), 90b, 93b, 112b, 114b–115b
  balance, 102
  intake, 71b
  prescription, 106
  restricted formulas, 137b
  restriction of, 143
Fluvastatin, 29b
folate, 81, 91b, 116b, 120, 149b
Folbee, 185
folic acid, 39b, 81, 82b, 100b, 185–186
food
  delivery, 133–135, 134b–135b, 136b–138b
  history, 16, 16b–18b
  intake, 16b, 65, 124, 175
  log, 139
  medication interaction, 59b
  safety, 151b–152b
fosinopril (Monopril), 20b
Fosrenol, 25b
fruit intake, 73t, 75, 145t
furosemide (Lasix), 19b

gastrointestinal (GI) symptoms, 23b, 149b
Gemfibrozil, 29b
GFR. *See* glomerular filtration rate (GFR)
GI. *See* gastrointestinal (GI) symptoms
gingival hyperplasia, 149b
Gliclazide, 27b
Glimepiride, 27b
Glipizide, 27b
glomerular filtration rate (GFR), 2t, 85, 103
  estimated, 3–4, 81
Glucerna, 138b
glucose, 31b, 59b, 109b, 146b
  assessment, 35b
  control, 84, 102
  fasting, 39b
  formulas, 138b
  intolerance, 138b
  oxidation, 89
Glyburide, 27b
graft survival, 79
guanfacine, 22b

HbA1c. *See* hemoglobin A1c
HD. *See* hemodialysis (HD)
HDL. *See* high-density lipoprotein (HDL)
A Healthy Food Guide for People on Dialysis, 144
A Healthy Food Guide for People with CKD, 144
hematocrit, 40b
heme iron polypeptide (Proferrin), 148t
Hemocyte. *See* ferrous fumarate (Ferro-Sequels, Hemocyte, Nephro-Fer)
hemodialysis (HD), 10, 47b, 87, 106, 108, 144, 169
  catheter, 108
  conventional home, 111
  maintenance, 94–95
  nocturnal, 111
  nocturnal home, 111
  short daily home, 111
  treatment times, 111t
hemoglobin, 105
hemoglobin A1c (HbA1c), 4, 78, 97, 118
hemolysis (HD), 87, 106
high-density lipoprotein (HDL), 98b
hydralazine (Apresoline), 22b

hydrochlorothiazide (Microzide, HydroDiuril), 19*b*
HydroDiuril. *See* hydrochlorothiazide (Microzide, HydroDiuril)
hypercalcemia, 23*b*, 85, 103, 130
hyperglycemia, 78, 93*b*, 95, 118, 146*b*, 149*b*–150*b*
hyperhomocysteinemia, 82*b*, 120
hyperkalemia, 84, 102–103, 112*b*, 114*b*, 121, 149*b*–150*b*
hyperlipidemia, 149*b*–151*b*
hyperoxalosis, 81, 101, 119
hyperparathyroidism, 85, 104
hyperphosphatemia, 85, 103, 129
hypertension, 114*b*, 149*b*, 150*b*
hypoaldosteronism, 85
hypocholesterolemics, 31*b*
hypoglycemia, 27*b*, 78, 95, 109*b*, 118, 146*b*
hypokalemia, 84, 103, 112*b*, 121, 151*b*
hypomagnesemia, 149*b*–150*b*
hyponatremia, 129
hypophosphatemia, 116*b*, 121
hyporeninemia, 85
Hytrin. *See* terazosin (Hytrin)

IBW. *See* ideal body weight (IBW)
icodextrin, 143
ICU. *See* intensive care unit (ICU)
ideal body weight (IBW), 45*b*, 66
IDPN. *See* intradialytic parenteral nutrition (IDPN)
IG Tags. *See* Interpretative Guideline (IG) Tags
immediate-release verapamil (Calan, Isoptin), 21*b*
immunosuppressants, 148
Imuran. *See* azathioprine (Imuran)
incretin mimetics, 28*b*
indapamide (Lozol), 19*b*
Inderal. *See* propranolol (Inderal)
Inderal LA. *See* long-acting propranolol (Inderal LA)
infection, 149*b*
infectious morbidity, 111
inflammation assessment, 36*b*
Inspra. *See* eplerenone (Inspra)
insulin, 27*b*, 109*b*, 124
 resistance, 110
intake, 54

domain, 68, 178
intensive care unit (ICU), 110
Interpretative Guideline (IG) Tags, 9*b*
intradialytic parenteral nutrition (IDPN), 106–108, 108*b*
 macronutrients and electrolytes for, 109*b*
intraperitoneal amino acid (IPAA), 106, 110
intravenous fluids, 133, 135
intubation, 111
IPAA. *See* intraperitoneal amino acid (IPAA)
irbesartan (Avapro), 21*b*
iron, 71*b*. *See also* minerals
iron-deficiency anemia, 81, 119
iron polysaccharide complex (EzFe, Ferrex 150, Niferex, Niferex-150), 148*t*
isoniazid, 30*b*, 124
Isoptin. *See* immediate-release verapamil (Calan, Isoptin)
Isoptin SR. *See* long-acting verapamil (Calan SR, Isoptin SR)
Isosource, 136*b*
isradipine (Dynacirc CR), 21*b*

Jevity, 137*b*
Journal of Renal Nutrition, 140

K. *See* minerals; potassium (K)
KDIGO. *See* Kidney Disease Improving Global Outcomes (KDIGO)
KDOQI. *See* Kidney Disease Outcomes Quality Initiative (KDOQI)
Kerlone. *See* betaxolol (Kerlone)
ketoacid, oral, 77*t*
Ketorena, 77*t*
Ketosteril, 77*t*
kidney
 diet, 96
 failure, 2
 function assessment, 36*b*
 injury, acute, 47*b*
 physiology, 15
 transplant, 2, 79, 81, 121, 148
Kidney Disease Improving Global Outcomes (KDIGO), 2, 122

Kidney Disease Outcomes Quality Initiative (KDOQI), 1, 32, 74, 110, 118, 170
knowledge etiology, 63
K-Phos, 134b–135b

labetalol (Normodyne, Trandate), 20b
lansoprazole, 124
lanthanum carbonate, 24b–25b
Lasix. *See* furosemide (Lasix)
laxatives, 31b
LDL. *See* low-density lipoprotein (LDL)
Levatol. *See* penbutolol (Levatol)
Life Options program, 140b
lipids, 90b, 109b, 112b, 118
lipoproteins, 41b
lisinopril (Prinivil, Zestril), 20b
long-acting nifedipine (Adalat CC, Procardia XL), 21b
long-acting propranolol (Inderal LA), 20b
long-acting verapamil (Calan SR, Isoptin SR), 21b
Loniten. *See* minoxidil (Loniten)
loop diuretics, 19b
Lopressor. *See* metoprolol (Lopressor)
losartan (Cozaar), 21b
LoseIt, 139
Lotensin. *See* benazepril (Lotensin)
Lovastatin, 29b
low-density lipoprotein (LDL), 98b
Lozol. *See* indapamide (Lozol)

Maalox, 86, 105
macronutrients, 89b, 90b, 109b
Magnebind, 25b
magnesium, 41b, 86–88, 90b, 105, 109b, 114b, 116b
carbonate, 25b
Magonate, 25b
maintenance hemodialysis (MHD), 92, 93b–94b, 97b–98b
malabsorption, 137b
malnutrition, 60b, 95
manganese, 92b
Marinol. *See* dronabinol (Marinol)
Mavik. *See* trandolapril (Mavik)
MCT oil. *See* medium-chain triglyceride (MCT) oil

MCV. *See* mean corpuscular volume (MCV)
mean corpuscular volume (MCV), 42b, 81
medical diagnoses, 54
medical food supplement therapy, 133
medical nutrition therapy (MNT), 2–6, 4b, 5t, 139
  acute and chronic posttransplantation, 113, 114b–116b
  based on chronic kidney disease stage, 8–10, 9b
  for patients with CKD stage 1 through 4, 72, 72t–74t
  pretransplantation, 113
  recommendations, 93b–94b
  screening and referral for, 6–8, 7b
Medicare
  conditions for coverage, 9b
  COVID-19 pandemic and, 6
  Part B, 5t, 5–6
medication(s), 65, 124. *See also specific medication*
  history, 19
Mediterranean diet, 75, 117
medium-chain triglyceride (MCT) oil, 136
MedLine Plus, 141b
megestrol acetate (Megace), 144b
Meglitinides, 28b
metabolically stable, 76b
metabolic stress, 95
Metformin, 28b
methyldopa (Aldomet), 22b
metolazone (Mykrox, Zaroxolyn), 19b
metoprolol (Lopressor), 20b
MHD. *See* maintenance hemodialysis (MHD)
Micardis. *See* telmisartan (Micardis)
micronutrient(s), 90b, 94b, 115b
  prescription, 79–80, 82b–83b, 99, 118–119
Microzide. *See* hydrochlorothiazide (Microzide, HydroDiuril)
Midamor. *See* amiloride (Midamor)
Miglitol, 27b
Milk of Magnesia, 86, 105
mineral oil, 31b

minerals
　　calcium (Ca), 23b–24b, 24b, 43b, 71b, 74t, 85–88, 90t, 94b, 103, 114b–116b, 121, 124, 147
　　iron, 40b, 71b, 81, 86, 101, 105, 119, 122, 147, 148t
　　phosphorus, 5, 22b–26b, 43b, 58b, 71b, 73t, 85–86, 88, 90b, 94b, 103–104, 104t, 109b–116b, 121–122, 127, 134b–135b, 145–147, 179
　　potassium (K), 5, 19b–20b, 31b, 58b–59b, 71b, 74t, 84–85, 88, 90b, 94b, 102–103, 109b, 112b, 114b, 116b, 120–121, 134b–135b
　　sodium, 71b, 73t, 83, 90b, 94b, 102, 112b, 114b, 116b, 120, 127, 134b–135b, 143, 149b
minerals, chronic kidney disease (CKD) and, 71b
mineral(s), 114b, 116b
　　intake, 58b, 71b
　　prescription, 102–106, 104t, 120–121
Minipress. *See* prazosin (Minipress)
minoxidil (Loniten), 22b
mirtazapine (Remeron), 144b
MNT. *See* medical nutrition therapy (MNT)
moexipril (Univasc), 20b
Monopril. *See* fosinopril (Monopril)
monounsaturated fat, 79, 97, 118
morbidity, 111
mortality, 97b, 103
mouth ulcers, 149b
multivitamin (MVI), 80, 91b, 94b, 99, 112b, 115, 124
muromonab-CD3 (Orthoclone OKT3), 150b
muscle mass, 117
MVI. *See* multivitamin (MVI)
mycophenolate, 30b
mycophenolate mofetil (Cellcept, RS-61443), 150b
MyFitnessPal, 139
Mykrox. *See* metolazone (Mykrox, Zaroxolyn)

nadolol (Corgard), 20b
nateglinide (28b)
National Heart, Lung, and Blood Institute, 144

National Kidney Diet, 140b
National Kidney Disease Education Program, 141b
National Kidney Foundation (NKF), 1, 141b
NCP. *See* Nutrition Care Process (NCP)
NCPT. *See Abridged Nutrition Care Process Terminology (NCPT) Reference Manual*; Nutrition Care Process Terminology (NCPT)
NEAP. *See* net acid production (NEAP)
neomycin, 30b
Neoral. *See* cyclosporine A (Sandimmune, Neoral)
NephPlexRx, 185
Nephrocap, 185
Nephro-Fer. *See* ferrous fumarate (Ferro-Sequels, Hemocyte, Nephro-Fer)
Nephronex, 185–186
nephrotic syndrome, 81
Nephro-Vite Rx, 185–186
Nepro, 138b
net acid production (NEAP), 75
neuropathy, 118
neurotoxicity, 105
NHD. *See* nocturnal hemodialysis (NHD)
NHHD. *See* nocturnal home hemodialysis (NHHD)
Niacin (vitamin B3), 29b, 82b, 91b, 100b, 185–186
Niferex. *See* iron polysaccharide complex (EzFe, Ferrex 150, Niferex, Niferex-150)
nisoldipine (Sular), 21b
nitrogen, 117
NKF. *See* National Kidney Foundation (NKF)
nocturnal hemodialysis (NHD), 111
nocturnal home hemodialysis (NHHD), 111
　　nutrition guidelines for, 112b
Nondihydropyridine, 21b
Normodyne. *See* labetalol (Normodyne, Trandate)
Norvasc. *See* amlodipine (Norvasc)
Nutren, 136b
　　2.0, 137b
　　with fiber, 137b

Index

nutrient(s)
  absorption and utilization of, 30*b*–31*b*, 59*b*
  delivery, 133–135, 134*b*–135*b*, 136*b*–138*b*
  intake of, 16*b*
  needs, 58*b*
nutrition
  ASPEN, 2
  assessment, 1, 15–16, 16*b*–31*b*, 18–19, 32–34, 33*b*–42*b*, 43–45, 43*t*, 45*b*–46*b*, 46*t*–47*t*, 48–51, 65–68, 71*b*, 124–126, 160–161, 173*b*, 175–178
  care manual, 140*b*
  case study, 48–51, 65–69
  coordination of care, 159
  counseling, 152–155, 153*b*–158*b*, 158–159, 167, 181
  diagnoses for CKD, 57*b*–60*b*, 71*b*
  diagnosis, 1, 54–56, 57*b*–62*b*, 62–69, 64*f*, 68–69, 127–128, 163–164, 173*b*, 178–179
  diagnosis etiology category identification, 62–63
  diagnosis reference sheet, 64, 64*f*
  documentation of, 170–171, 173*b*–174*b*
  education, 138–139, 140*b*–144*b*, 143–148, 145*t*, 146*b*, 148*t*, 149*b*–152b, 166, 181
  enteral, 71*b*
  evaluation, 1
  5 A's in, 152–155, 153*b*–158*b*, 158–159
  intervention, 1, 128–129, 164–166, 173*b*, 179–181
  laboratory data, 50, 59*b*, 67
  monitoring and evaluation of, 1, 169–171, 171*b*–174*b*, 174–182
  for nocturnal home hemodialysis, 112*b*
  parenteral, 71*b*
  physical findings, 43–44
  prescription, 70, 71*b*, 92, 93*b*–94*b*, 94–95, 113, 114*b*–116*b*, 117–123, 129
  supplementation, 87–89, 88*t*–89*t*, 89*b*–92*b*, 106–111, 109*b*, 122–123, 133
Nutrition Care Model, 54
Nutrition Care Process (NCP), 1, 15, 54, 70, 169
  case study, 123–129, 160–167, 174–182
  steps of, 3*b*

Nutrition Care Process Terminology (NCPT), 54, 70
nutrition intervention
  implementation, 133–135, 134*b*–138*b*, 138–139, 140*b*–144*b*, 143–148, 145*t*, 146*b*, 148*b*–158*b*, 152–155, 158–167
  prescription planning, 70–72, 71*b*, 72*t*–74*t*, 74–81, 76*b*, 77*t*, 82*b*–83*b*, 83–89, 88*t*–89*t*, 89*b*–94*b*, 92, 94–97, 96*t*, 97*b*–98*b*, 99, 100*b*, 101–108, 104*t*, 109*b*, 110–113, 111*t*, 112*b*, 114*b*–116*b*, 117–129

obesity, 34*b*
olmesartan (Benicar), 21*b*
omega-3 polyunsaturated fatty acid (PUFA), 93*b*, 97, 97*b*
ONS. *See* oral nutritional supplementation (ONS)
oral intake, 57*b*
oral nutritional supplementation (ONS), 87, 106–108, 123, 136*b*
Orthoclone OKT3. *See* muromonab-CD3 (Orthoclone OKT3)
Osmolite, 136*b*
osteomalacia, 105

pantothenic acid (vitamin B5), 83*b*, 91*b*, 100*b*, 185–186
parathyroid hormone (PTH), 23*b*, 40*b*, 43*b*, 85
parenteral nutrition (PN), 71*b*, 87, 123, 133, 135
  fat emulsions for, 89*t*
  prescription, 88, 88*t*, 110–111
  solution, 89*b*–92*b*
patient history, 44, 68, 126, 163, 178
PD. *See* peritoneal dialysis (PD)
penbutolol (Levatol), 20*b*
Peptamen, 137*b*
peptide-based formulas, 137*b*
perindopril (Aceon), 20*b*
peritoneal dialysate solution, 96
peritoneal dialysis (PD), 5, 10, 92*b*–98*b*, 95, 128, 143–144, 169
  dextrose contribution of, 96*t*
  regimen, 164–166, 179–181
peritonitis, 95, 128

PES statement. *See* problem, etiology, signs and symptoms (PES) statement
PEW. *See* protein-energy wasting (PEW)
Phillips' Milk of Magnesia, 86, 105
PhosLo, 23*b*
Phoslyra, 23*b*
Phos-NaK powder, 134*b*
Phospha 250 Neutral, 135*b*
phosphorus, 71*b*. *See also* minerals
physical activity
  guidelines, 142*b*–143*b*
  tracker applications, 139
physical therapy, 143
physiologic-metabolic etiology, 63
pioglitazone, 28*b*
plan of care (POC), 9*b*
Plendil. *See* felodipine (Plendil)
PN. *See* parenteral nutrition (PN)
POC. *See* plan of care (POC)
polythiazide (Renese), 19*b*
polyunsaturated fat, 79, 97, 118
polyunsaturated fatty acids (PUFA), 79
posttransplantation, 4, 10, 113
potassium (K), 71*b*. *See also* minerals
pramlintide, 28*b*
pravastatin, 29*b*
prazosin (Minipress), 22*b*
prealbumin, 42*b*
prednisolone, 149*b*–150*b*
Prednisone, 149*b*–150*b*
Prinivil. *See* lisinopril (Prinivil, Zestril)
problem, etiology, signs and symptoms (PES) statement, 55–56, 68–70, 127, 179
Procardia XL. *See* long-acting nifedipine (Adalat CC, Procardia XL)
Proferrin. *See* heme iron polypeptide (Proferrin)
Prograf. *See* tacrolimus (Prograf, FK506)
propranolol (Inderal), 20*b*
ProRenal+D, 186
protein, 58*b*, 72*t*, 93*b*, 112*b*, 114*b*–115*b*, 128
  catabolism, 150*b*
  diet, 76
  energy malnutrition, 36*b*
  intake, 84, 95, 102, 144–146, 145*t*, 146*b*
  modulars, 136*b*
  needs, 71*b*
  prescription, 75–76, 92, 117

protein-energy wasting (PEW), 76, 87, 106, 122
proteinuria, 83
psychological etiology, 63
PTH. *See* parathyroid hormone (PTH)
PUFA. *See* omega-3 polyunsaturated fatty acid (PUFA); polyunsaturated fatty acids (PUFA)
Pure Protein Bars, 136*b*
pyridoxine (vitamin B6), 82*b*, 91*b*, 100*b*, 185–186

ramipril (Altace), 20*b*
Rapamune. *See* sirolimus (Rapamune)
RDA. *See* Recommended Dietary Allowance (RDA)
RDN. *See* registered dietitian nutritionist (RDN)
Recommended Dietary Allowance (RDA), 79–80, 99, 119
registered dietitian nutritionist (RDN), 4, 6, 32, 54, 75, 99, 139
Remeron. *See* mirtazapine (Remeron)
Renagel, 26*b*
renal bone disease, 85, 104. *See also* kidney
Renalcal, 138*b*
renal diet, 96
Renal Dietitians Dietetic Practice Group of the Academy of Nutrition and Dietetics, 141*b*
renal failure. *See* kidney
renal replacement therapy (RRT), 6
Renal Tab, 186
renal transplant, 79, 81, 148. *See also* kidney
RenaPlex, 186
Rena-Vite, 186
Renese. *See* polythiazide (Renese)
Reno Caps, 185
Renvela, 26*b*
Repaglinide, 28*b*
reserpine, 22*b*
retinopathy, 118
riboflavin (vitamin B2), 82*b*, 91*b*, 100*b*, 185–186
rosiglitazone, 28*b*
rosuvastatin, 29*b*
RRT. *See* renal replacement therapy (RRT)

RS-61443. *See* mycophenolate mofetil (Cellcept, RS-61443)

Sandimmune. *See* cyclosporine A (Sandimmune, Neoral)
saturated fat, 73*t*, 79, 93*b*, 97, 118
Sectral. *See* acebutolol (Sectral)
selenium, 83*b*, 87, 92*b*, 106, 185–186
self-monitoring deficit, 61*b*
serum transferrin saturation (TSAT), 86, 122
sevelamer, 124
 carbonate, 25*b*
 hydrochloride, 26*b*
short daily home hemodialysis, 111
Simulect. *See* basiliximab (Simulect)
simvastatin, 29*b*
sirolimus (Rapamune), 151*b*
sitagliptin, 28*b*
skeletal myopathy, 87, 106
Slow Fe. *See* ferrous sulfate (Feosol, Slow Fe)
social-personal etiology, 63
sodium, 71*b*. *See also* minerals
Sodium Glucose Cotransporter 2 Inhibitors, 28*b*
soft tissue calcification, 85, 103–104
soluble fiber, 73*t*
Solu-Medrol, 149*b*–150*b*
spironolactone (Aldactone, CaroSpir), 19*b*, 31*b*
standard body weight, 46*b*
statins, 29*b*, 124
sucroferric oxyhydroxide, 26*b*
Sular. *See* nisoldipine (Sular)
sulfonylureas, 27*b*
Suplena, 138*b*

tacrolimus (Prograf, FK506), 31*b*, 150*b*
telmisartan (Micardis), 21*b*
Tenormin. *See* atenolol (Tenormin)
terazosin (Hytrin), 22*b*
tetracycline, 30*b*
Teveten. *See* eprosartan (Teveten)
TG. *See* triglyceride (TG)
Thiamin (vitamin B1), 82*b*, 91*b*, 100*b*, 124, 185–186
thiazides, 19*b*

thiazolidinediones, 28*b*
thyroid dysfunction, 87, 106
Tiazac. *See* extended-release diltiazem (Cardizem CD, Dilacor XR, Tiazac, Cardizem LA)
timolol (Blocadren), 20*b*
tobramycin, 30*b*
tolazamide, 27*b*
tolbutamide, 27*b*
Toprol XL. *See* extended-release metoprolol (Toprol XL)
torsemide (Dyrenium), 19*b*
total fat, 73*t*, 93*b*
trace elements, 91*b*–92*b*
Trandate. *See* labetalol (Normodyne, Trandate)
trandolapril (Mavik), 20*b*
trans fat, 79, 97, 118
transferrin, 105
triamterene (Dyrenium), 19*b*
triglyceride (TG), 98*b*, 109*b*, 112*b*
TSAT. *See* serum transferrin saturation (TSAT)
TUMS, 23*b*
25-hydroxyvitamin D serum level, 80, 101, 119
TwoCal HN, 137*b*

Univasc. *See* moexipril (Univasc)

valsartan (Diovan), 21*b*
vasodilators, 22*b*
Vasotec. *See* enalapril (Vasotec)
vegetable intake, 73*t*, 75, 145*t*
Velphoro, 26*b*
Verelan PM. *See* extended-release verapamil hydrochloride (Covera HS, Verelan PM)
Vital-D Rx, 185
vitamin B1. *See* Thiamin (vitamin B1)
vitamin B2. *See* Riboflavin (vitamin B2)
vitamin B3. *See* Niacin (vitamin B3)
vitamin B5. *See* pantothenic acid (vitamin B5); Pantothenic acid (vitamin B5)
vitamin B6. *See* Pyridoxine (vitamin B6)
vitamin B12. *See* cobalamin (vitamin B12); cyanocobalamin (vitamin B12)

vitamin D2. *See* ergocalciferol (vitamin D2)
vitamin D3. *See* cholecalciferol (vitamin D3)
vitamin(s), 114*b*
  A, 80, 82*b*, 91*b*, 100*b*, 101
  B, 147
  C, 58*b*, 81–82, 91*b*, 100–101, 116*b*, 119, 147, 185–186
  D, 80, 82*b*, 85–86, 91*b*, 94*b*, 100–104, 116*b*, 119, 148
  D analogs, 103
  E, 82*b*, 91*b*, 100*b*, 101, 185–186
  intake, 58*b*, 71*b*, 80
  K, 82*b*, 91*b*, 100*b*, 116*b*
  prescription, 80–81, 82*b*–83*b*, 99, 100*b*, 101, 119–120
  recommendations, 100*b*
  renal-specific, 184–186
  toxicity, 99, 101
  water-soluble, 99, 112*b*
Vivonex, 137*b*

warfarin, 116*b*, 119
water-soluble vitamins, 99, 112*b*
weight
  adjusted body, 45*b*–46*b*
  body weight (BW), 32, 45*b*–46*b*, 60*b*, 75, 93*b*
  edema-free, 46*b*
  estimated dry weight (EDW), 66
  gain, 60*b*, 96, 142*b*, 143, 144*b*
  ideal body weight (IBW), 45*b*, 66
  loss, 60*b*, 139, 140*b*–143*b*, 143
  maintenance, 142*b*
  management, 139, 140*b*–144*b*, 143
  program, 143
  standard body, 46*b*
wound, 151*b*

Zaroxolyn. *See* metolazone (Mykrox, Zaroxolyn)
Zebeta. *See* bisoprolol (Zebeta)
Zenapax. *See* daclizumab (Zenapax)
Zestril. *See* lisinopril (Prinivil, Zestril)
zinc, 83*b*, 86–87, 91*b*, 105–106, 185–186
ZonePerfect Bars, 136*b*